AF774509

Controversies in Pediatric and Adolescent Hematology

Pediatric and Adolescent Medicine

Vol. 17

Series Editors

David Branski Jerusalem
Wieland Kiess Leipzig

Controversies in Pediatric and Adolescent Hematology

Volume Editors

Angela E. Thomas Edinburgh
Christina Halsey Glasgow

13 figures, and 19 tables, 2014

KARGER

Basel · Freiburg · Paris · London · New York · New Delhi · Bangkok · Beijing · Tokyo · Kuala Lumpur · Singapore · Sydney

Pediatric and Adolescent Medicine
Founded 1991 by D. Branski, Jerusalem

Angela E. Thomas
Consultant Pediatric Hematologist
Royal Hospital for Sick Children
Edinburgh
EH9 1LF

Christina Halsey
Consultant Pediatric Hematologist and
Scottish Senior Clinical Research Fellow
Institute of Infection, Immunity and
Inflammation
College of Medical, Veterinary and Life Sciences
University of Glasgow
Glasgow
G12 8TA

Library of Congress Cataloging-in-Publication Data

Controversies in pediatric and adolescent hematology / volume editors, Angela E. Thomas, Christina Halsey.
p. ; cm. -- (Pediatric and adolescent medicine, ISSN 1017-5989 ; vol. 17)
Includes bibliographical references and indexes.
ISBN 978-3-318-02422-7 (hard cover : alk. paper) -- ISBN (invalid) 978-3-318-02423-4 (electronic version)
I. Thomas, Angela E., editor of compilation. II. Halsey, Christina, editor of compilation. III. Series: Pediatric and adolescent medicine ; v. 17. 1017-5989
[DNLM: 1. Child. 2. Hematologic Diseases. 3. Adolescent. 4. Infant. W1 PE163HL v.17 2014 / WS 300]
RJ269.5
618.92'15--dc23

2013034474

Bibliographic Indices. This publication is listed in bibliographic services, including Current Contents®.

Disclaimer. The statements, opinions and data contained in this publication are solely those of the individual authors and contributors and not of the publisher and the editor(s). The appearance of advertisements in the book is not a warranty, endorsement, or approval of the products or services advertised or of their effectiveness, quality or safety. The publisher and the editor(s) disclaim responsibility for any injury to persons or property resulting from any ideas, methods, instructions or products referred to in the content or advertisements.

Drug Dosage. The authors and the publisher have exerted every effort to ensure that drug selection and dosage set forth in this text are in accord with current recommendations and practice at the time of publication. However, in view of ongoing research, changes in government regulations, and the constant flow of information relating to drug therapy and drug reactions, the reader is urged to check the package insert for each drug for any change in indications and dosage and for added warnings and precautions. This is particularly important when the recommended agent is a new and/or infrequently employed drug.

All rights reserved. No part of this publication may be translated into other languages, reproduced or utilized in any form or by any means electronic or mechanical, including photocopying, recording, microcopying, or by any information storage and retrieval system, without permission in writing from the publisher.

© Copyright 2014 by S. Karger AG, P.O. Box, CH–4009 Basel (Switzerland)
www.karger.com
Printed in Germany on acid-free and non-aging paper (ISO 9706) by Kraft Druck GmbH, Ettlingen
ISSN 1017–5989
e-ISSN 1662–3886
ISBN 978–3–318–02422–7
e-ISBN 978–3–318–02423–4

Contents

Preface

The care of infants, children and young people with hematological disorders provides a fascinating and ever changing spectrum of diagnoses, management challenges and treatment dilemmas. In infancy not only does the blood system undergo physiological changes in adaptation to the extra-uterine environment but it is also the time when congenital disease will present often for the first time within a family. During early childhood periods of rapid growth put great nutritional demands on the body and iron deficiency anemia is very common. Throughout childhood, the establishment of an immune repertoire with rapid lymphocyte proliferation in response to infectious challenge may also predispose to autoimmune disorders such as ITP or malignancies such as acute lymphoblastic leukemia. However, it is not only young children that provide challenges – adolescence is a time of great upheaval and there is increasing recognition of the unique needs of patients with lifelong conditions during their transition from pediatric to adult-centered models of care. In this volume, we focus on recent advances in the understanding and treatment of many of these neonatal, childhood and adolescent disorders. We are also delighted to include a chapter on the management of problems that may arise in the intensive care unit – either due to life-threatening presentations of primary hematological disorders or due to hematological responses secondary to significant systemic illness.

Drug therapy for pediatric disorders is particularly challenging, many drugs are unlicensed in children and it is often difficult to extrapolate optimal treatment schedules from adult data. In addition, although children often tolerate toxic treatment for conditions such as leukemia much better than adults, the impact of late effects of treatment can be much greater due to the long life expectancy. This leads to great debate and controversy: How aggressive does the treatment need to be? What are the long-term effects of treatment? Can we tailor treatment more specifically to individuals to maximize benefit while minimizing risk? These questions are addressed in this volume for a spectrum of diseases with some of the controversies moving towards resolution, for the time being at least, and translating into advances in clinical practise.

We are very grateful to the authors for their expertise and enthusiasm in helping us complete this project in a timely fashion and to the publishers for their help and encouragement with the volume. We hope that you both enjoy the debate and discussion in the book and find it a useful tool for your clinical practise.

Angela E. Thomas, Edinburgh
Christina Halsey, Glasgow

Thomas AE, Halsey C (eds): Controversies in Pediatric and Adolescent Hematology.
Pediatr Adolesc Med. Basel, Karger, 2014, vol 17, pp 1–15 (DOI: 10.1159/000350343)

Neonatal Thrombocytopenia

Subarna Chakravorty · Irene Roberts

Centre for Haematology, Imperial College London and Department of Paediatrics, St Mary's Hospital, Imperial College Healthcare NHS Trust, London, UK

Abstract

Thrombocytopenia is the commonest haematological abnormality in neonates where the advice of a haematologist is sought and specialist management may be necessary to prevent associated mortality or long-term disability. The majority of neonates who present with thrombocytopenia within 72 h of birth are preterm and born to mothers with placental dysfunction where chronic fetal hypoxia perturbs normal platelet production. In such cases, thrombocytopenia is usually mild to moderate (platelets 50–150 × 10^9/l) and resolves within 10 days of birth. Neonatal thrombocytopenia presenting after 72 h of age is usually due to late-onset sepsis or necrotising enterocolitis and is frequently severe and treated with multiple platelet transfusions. In term neonates, where thrombocytopenia is much less common, the clinically most important cause is neonatal alloimmune thrombocytopenia (NAIT). Around 10% of children with NAIT develop intracranial haemorrhage, which may occur prior to birth. Prompt diagnosis and transfusion of HPA-compatible platelets is key to successful management of NAIT. Recent studies indicate that many neonates with severe thrombocytopenia receive platelet transfusions based on consensus national or local guidelines despite little evidence of benefit. Controlled trials of platelet transfusion for neonatal thrombocytopenia, currently in progress, are needed to improve the management of this common complication of neonatal medicine.

Copyright © 2014 S. Karger AG, Basel

Neonatal thrombocytopenia, whilst rare in the general population, is frequently encountered in neonatal intensive care units, particularly among very low birth weight or sick neonates, up to 80% of which may be affected [1, 2]. Thrombocytopenia usually occurs as a response to a systemic disorder, and in most cases, resolves spontaneously or following resolution of the underlying pathology. However, the risk of significant or serious haemorrhage in thrombocytopenic neonates is high [3], particularly in those who are very preterm or have low birth weight. The treatment of thrombocytopenia, particularly in the context of platelet transfusion thresholds, remains controversial, and lacks consensus among neonatologists around the world [4].

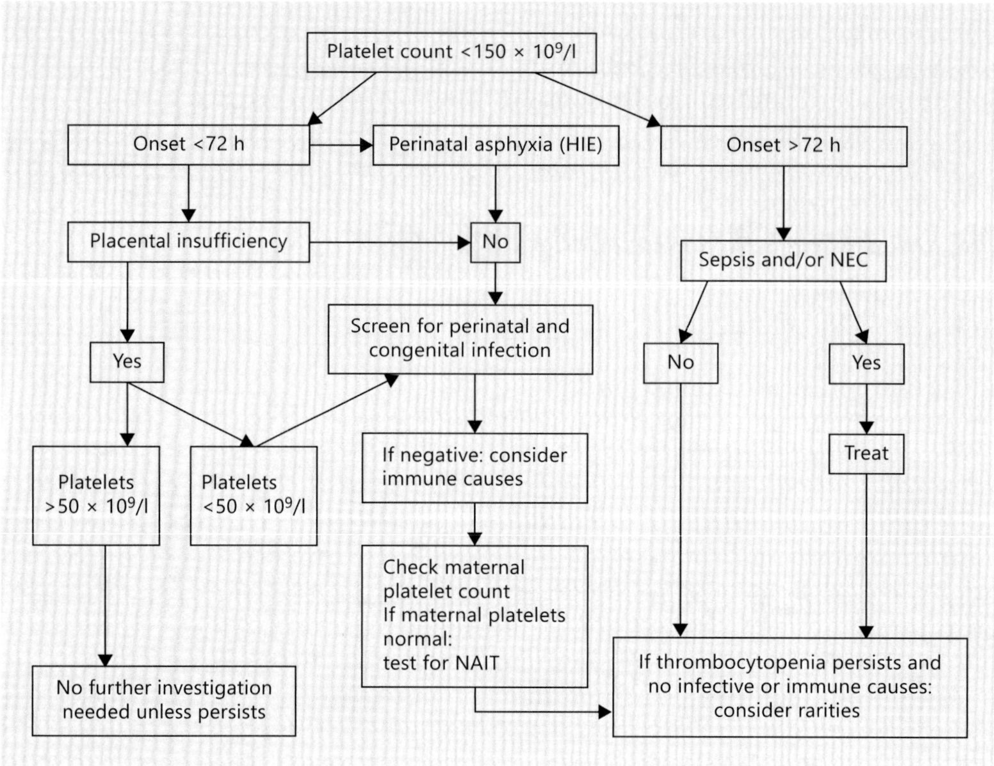

Fig. 1. Diagnostic algorithm for neonatal thrombocytopenia in preterm neonates.

In the majority of patients, thrombocytopenia resolves spontaneously with few long-term sequelae, so expensive and time-consuming investigations are usually not necessary, provided a clinical diagnostic algorithm is followed (fig. 1, 2). In practice, this can be achieved by stratifying the causes of thrombocytopenia according to the post-natal age of the neonate at presentation and the gestational age and weight at birth, all of which can guide the clinician in making the right clinical and investigative choices. The risk of bleeding in thrombocytopenic neonates is higher in severe thrombocytopenia (generally considered to be a platelet count of $<50 \times 10^9$/l), and the majority of diagnostic and therapeutic interventions are aimed at preventing such events, which may be catastrophic and result in severe disability or death [5].

In this chapter we discuss how neonatal thrombopoiesis differs from that of adults, and how this may be reflected in the clinical presentation and management of neonatal thrombocytopenia. We also discuss the incidence of neonatal thrombocytopenia in term and preterm infants and the causes and natural history of thrombocytopenia depending upon the age at presentation and the duration and severity of thrombocytopenia. Finally, we discuss current therapeutic options, including the role of platelet transfusion, and suggest a practical therapeutic and diagnostic algorithm to help clinicians with management of thrombocytopenia in the neonate (fig. 1, 2).

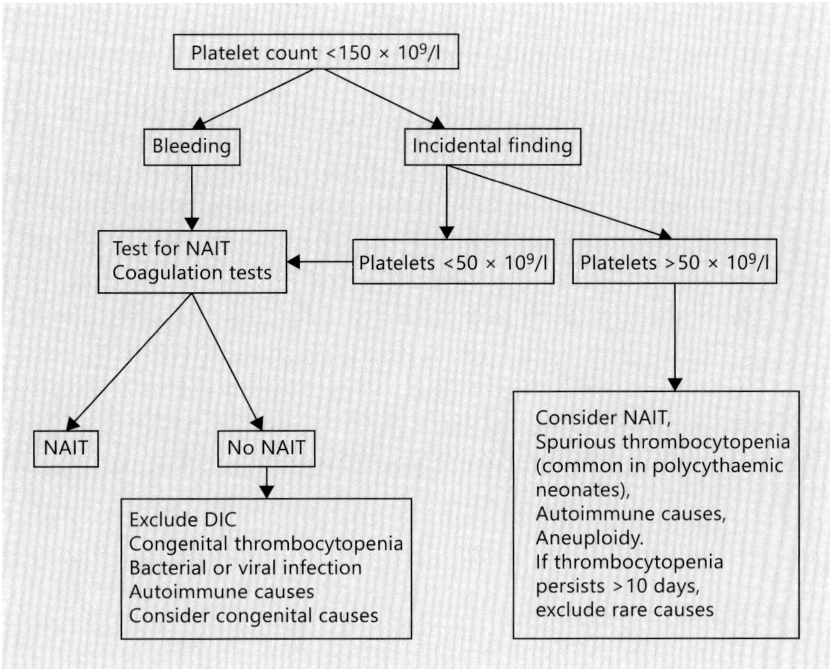

Fig. 2. Diagnostic algorithm for neonatal thrombocytopenia in term neonates.

Thrombopoiesis in the Fetus and Neonate

Platelets appear in the fetal circulation as early as the 5th week of post-conceptual age and reach values of 150×10^9/l by the end of the first trimester [6]. Therefore, all viable fetuses with platelet counts of $<150 \times 10^9$/l can be considered thrombocytopenic. This definition was recently challenged by a retrospective analysis of 47,000 neonates, where a reference range of platelet counts at different gestational ages was determined by excluding the highest and lowest 5th percentile of all observed counts. By this method, the lowest limit of platelet counts for infants <32 weeks' gestation was found to be 104×10^9/l, compared to 123×10^9/l for neonates >32 weeks' gestation [7]. However, as the study included all neonates, regardless of clinical status, these counts may simply reflect what is normally observed in neonatal units, rather than what might be considered a new physiological definition of normal platelet counts in the newborn. Indeed, the mean platelet count was $>200 \times 10^9$/l regardless of gestation at birth, reflecting what was already known about platelet reference ranges in neonates.

There is now a large body of evidence to indicate that fetal thrombopoiesis differs from that of adults [8, 9]. Reticulated (young) platelets are more numerous in the fetus compared with adults, and fetal megakaryocytes are smaller and of lower ploidy compared with their adult counterparts [9]. Despite this, fetal megakaryocytes appear to be cytoplasmically mature and express increased amounts of GATA1 and surface glycoprotein 1b compared with those of adults. Additionally, fetal megakaryocytes have more proliferative potential in vitro than those derived from adults and are more sensitive to thrombopoietin, and circulating thrombopoietin levels in healthy neonates are higher than those in adults, indicating that despite the megakaryocytes being smaller, fetal and neonatal platelet counts are maintained at levels similar to that of adults by virtue of their greater proliferative potential [8]. There are also developmental differences in megakaryocyte progenitor cells. Firstly, the numbers of megakaryocyte progenitors (burst-forming units-megakaryocyte and colony-forming units-megakaryocyte) and megakaryocytes are high early in fetal life and fall towards term and are higher in healthy preterm than term babies [8]. Furthermore, thrombocytopenic neonates, unlike adults, can only increase their megakaryocyte number, and not size, in response to consumptive thrombocytopenia [10]. Taken together, these data highlight the fundamental differences in adult and neonatal thrombopoiesis, which are important to consider when investigating and treating neonatal thrombocytopenia.

Incidence of Neonatal Thrombocytopenia

Thrombocytopenia is the commonest haematological abnormality detected in neonates. Depending on the population studied, platelet counts of $<150 \times 10^9$/l can be found in 1–5% of neonates overall and 0.1–0.5% of neonates present with severe thrombocytopenia (platelets $<50 \times 10^9$/l) [11]. The incidence of thrombocytopenia increases significantly in neonates who are admitted to neonatal intensive care units (NICU), where thrombocytopenia can occur in ~40% of all patients. The severity of thrombocytopenia worsens with prematurity and severity of clinical condition: the incidence of thrombocytopenia in sick neonates requiring intensive care can be as high as 70–80% [1].

Clinical Classification of Neonatal Thrombocytopenia

Although thrombocytopenia may have a wide variety of causes, clinical presentation of neonatal thrombocytopenia can broadly be divided into three groups depending on the age at presentation, regardless of aetiology:

- fetal thrombocytopenia,
- thrombocytopenia presenting at <72 h age,
- thrombocytopenia presenting at >72 h of age.

The most common causes of thrombocytopenia presenting in the first 72 h of life, and occasionally in fetal life, are almost all related to complications of pregnancy and/or delivery (table 1). By contrast, the vast majority of neonates developing thrombocytopenia after the first 72 h of life do so as a result of a post-natally acquired bacterial infection and/or necrotizing enterocolitis (table 1).

Table 1. Classification of neonatal thrombocytopenia

Fetal	*Alloimmune- due to anti-HPA antibodies** *Congenital infection (e.g. CMV, Parvovirus, toxoplasma, rubella, HIV)* Aneuploidy (e.g. trisomies 18, 13, 21, or triploidy) Autoimmune (e.g. maternal immune thrombocytopenia, SLE) Severe haemolytic disease of the newborn (usually anti-Rh antibodies) Congenital/inherited (e.g. Bernard Soulier syndrome, congenital amegakaryocytic thrombocytopenia)
Early-onset neonatal (<72 h)	*Placental insufficiency (e.g. IUGR, PIH or diabetes)** *Hypoxic ischaemic encephalopathy ± whole body cooling** Perinatal infection (e.g. *E. coli*, Group B *Streptococcus, H. influenzae*) Disseminated intravascular coagulation Alloimmune Autoimmune (maternal immune thrombocytopenia, neonatal lupus) Congenital infection (as above) Trisomy 21-associated TMD; and other trisomies (e.g. trisomy 13 or 18) Thrombosis (Thrombotic Thrombocytopenic Purpura, renal vein thrombosis, heparin-induced thrombocytopenia) Bone marrow replacement (e.g. congenital leukaemia, osteopetrosis) Kasabach Merritt syndrome Metabolic disease (e.g. propionic and methylmalonic acidaemia) Congenital/inherited (as above)
Late-onset neonatal (>72 h)	*Late-onset sepsis- usually bacterial, may be fungal** *Necrotising enterocolitis** Viral/protozoal infection (e.g. CMV, toxoplasma, rubella, HIV, parvovirus), autoimmune, Kasabach Merritt syndrome Metabolic disease (e.g. propionic and methylmalonic acidaemia) Congenital/inherited (e.g. Bernard Soulier syndrome, congenital amegakaryocytic thrombocytopenia)

* Commonest causes in italics. CMV = Cytomegalovirus; HIV = human immune deficiency virus; HPA = human platelet antigen; IUGR = intrauterine growth restriction; PIH = pregnancy induced hypertension; SLE = systemic lupus erythematosus; TMD = transient myeloproliferative disorder.

This classification provides clinicians with guidance for selecting appropriate investigations and management and avoids unnecessary or expensive tests in transient thrombocytopenias where prognosis can be determined by simple clinical and laboratory means alone (fig. 1, 2; and discussion below).

Fetal Thrombocytopenia

Fetal thrombocytopenia is usually identified when fetal blood sampling is performed in cases where there is a known history of alloimmune thrombocytopenia or of inherited thrombocytopenia. Other cases of fetal thrombocytopenia present following fetal blood sampling for suspected fetal anomalies or fetal anaemia. Thus, the most common causes of fetal thrombocytopenia will be influenced by the particular case-mix of the Fetal Medicine Unit but include alloimmune thrombocytopenia, viral infection and thrombocytopenia secondary to severe alloimmune anaemia due to Rh alloantibodies.

Early-Onset Neonatal Thrombocytopenia (<72 h)

Three-quarters of all episodes of thrombocytopenia in patients admitted to NICU occur within the first 72 h of life. The majority of early-onset thrombocytopenias in the NICU occur in preterm neonates born to pregnancies complicated by placental insufficiency and/or chronic fetal hypoxia, secondary either to maternal disease (pregnancy-induced hypertension, hypertension, diabetes or HELLP (haemolysis, elevated liver enzymes and low platelets)) syndrome or to idiopathic intrauterine growth restriction in the fetus. The natural history of this type of neonatal thrombocytopenia is characteristic. Affected neonates often have a low normal or modestly reduced platelet count at birth ($120–200 \times 10^9$/l), which falls to a nadir of 80–100 at day 4–5 of life before recovering to $>150 \times 10^9$/l by 7–10 days of age. The presence of characteristic haematological features in routine blood films, including increased circulating erythroblasts, mild neutropenia, and often red cell changes of hyposplenism accompanying the thrombocytopenia, help make the diagnosis [12]. Indeed, if these features are present and the platelet count remains above 50×10^9/l and recovers with the characteristic natural history outlined above, no further investigations are necessary. On the other hand, if the platelet count falls below 50×10^9/l or thrombocytopenia persists beyond the 10th day of life, additional causes for the thrombocytopenia should be sought.

In contrast to the mild-to-moderate thrombocytopenia seen in most cases of placental insufficiency, early-onset severe thrombocytopenia ($<50 \times 10^9$/l) requires urgent investigation. The two most important causes are neonatal alloimmune thrombocytopenia (NAIT), which is discussed in detail below, and hypoxic ischaemic encephalopathy due to acute perinatal asphyxia/hypoxia. Up to 30% of all neonates with hypoxic ischaemic encephalopathy develop thrombocytopenia which is often severe and prolonged and principally appears to be precipitated by disseminated intravascular coagulation (DIC) [13].

Late-Onset Neonatal Thrombocytopenia (>72 h)

Late-onset thrombocytopenia in preterm neonates in the NICU is often severe, develops acutely and may be prolonged. The vast majority of late-onset thrombocytopenias are secondary to sepsis or necrotising enterocolitis (NEC). Many, but not all neonates with sepsis- or NEC-associated thrombocytopenia have evidence of DIC and so it is important to carry out a coagulation screen, including measurement of fibrinogen levels. Importantly, thrombocytopenia may be prolonged for several weeks beyond the onset of sepsis/NEC. Sepsis- and NEC-associated thrombocytopenia is one of the commonest indications for neonatal platelet transfusion [14].

Conditions Leading to Significant Thrombocytopenia in the Neonate

Although the majority of cases of neonatal thrombocytopenia can be diagnosed by their clinical presentation and basic laboratory parameters, there is a small number of conditions that lead to clinically significant thrombocytopenia and require specific investigation and management.

Neonatal Alloimmune Thrombocytopenia

NAIT is the commonest cause of severe thrombocytopenia in well, term infants and is caused by maternal sensitisation to paternally derived fetal antigens. Population-based studies indicate a prevalence of 0.7 per 1,000 pregnancies [15]. In Caucasian populations, human platelet antigen HPA1a is implicated in 80% cases of NAIT, and HPA5b in 10–15% [15]. The development of antibodies against HPA-1a in HPA-1a-negative women is strongly associated with HLA DRB3 0101 (OR 140). The laboratory diagnosis of NAIT is usually made using MAIPA (monoclonal antibody-specific immobilization of platelet antigens) assays to detect maternal anti-HPA antibodies. Both parents where possible and the infant should also be genotyped for the most common HPA alloantigens (HPA-1a, HPA-2, HPA-3, HPA-5b, and HPA-15). Unfortunately, in about 80% of neonates presenting with clinical features of NAIT, no antibodies or maternal-neonatal platelet incompatibility to these five HPA antigens is demonstrable. Very few of these unexplained cases have been shown to be due to antibodies against minor HPA (such as HPA-6w and HPA-9w) and, therefore, most groups do not recommend routine screening for these very-low-frequency HPA antigens in unexplained NAIT except in selected severe cases [16].

Most neonates with NAIT present with severe thrombocytopenia, often $<20 \times 10^9/l$. The most feared complication is intracranial haemorrhage (ICH) which occurs in ~20% of neonates with HPA1a-associated NAIT and is associated with a very high risk of severe neurodevelopmental problems, including cerebral palsy [5]. A high proportion of ICH (~80%) occurs in utero and NAIT has been reported as early as 20 weeks' gestation [15]. Since NAIT can affect first pregnancies, the diagnosis at birth is often unsuspected and the clinical presentation varies from asymptomatic thrombocytopenia or petechiae to seizures secondary to ICH.

Management of NAIT

All cases of suspected NAIT should undergo cranial ultrasound scans to exclude ICH. Most cases of NAIT resolve within a week without long-term sequelae. Since the platelet count usually falls over the first 4–7 days of life, all thrombocytopenic neonates with NAIT should be monitored until there is a sustained rise in their platelet count into the normal range. In well neonates with documented or suspected NAIT who have no evidence of haemorrhage, transfusion of HPA-compatible platelets is recommended only when the platelet count is $<30 \times 10^9$/l [17]. Usually, HPA-1a/5b-negative platelets are given pending an accurate diagnosis. In the event of major haemorrhage, including ICH, the platelet count should be maintained at $>50 \times 10^9$/l using appropriate HPA-negative platelets. In the UK HPA-1a/5b-negative platelets are available for immediate transfusion in most centres. However, when appropriate HPA-negative platelets are unobtainable, random donor platelet transfusions or intravenous immunoglobulin (IVIG) can be used in an emergency [17, 18]. In all cases, such platelets should be cytomegalovirus (CMV) antigen-negative and single-donor apheresis units; neonates who have received intrauterine platelet transfusions should be given irradiated platelets [19]. In some cases, thrombocytopenia may persist for up to 8–12 weeks. In these cases, IVIG is usually a better option than repeated platelet transfusions [1].

Antenatal Management of NAIT

At present, there is no consensus regarding best antenatal management of NAIT [recently reviewed in 18]. However, the most important point is that mothers of affected neonates should all be managed in subsequent pregnancies by fetal medicine units experienced in NAIT. Management of women with known HPA antibodies depends on the severity of previously affected neonates with NAIT, the HPA genotype of the father and on the HPA antibody specificity [18]. Although there is some evidence that antibody titres correlate with disease severity, the single most important predictor of poor outcome is a past history of an affected infant with ICH [17]. The optimal management of pregnancies at risk of NAIT is still unclear but most centres now rely mainly on risk-adapted, non-invasive strategies (an expectant 'wait and see' approach, at least in low risk cases, or administration of IVIG, with or without steroids, to the mother) in view of the procedure-associated risks of serial intrauterine platelet transfusions [reviewed in 17, 18].

Neonatal Autoimmune Thrombocytopenia

Transplacental passage of maternal platelet autoantibodies due to maternal immune thrombocytopenia or SLE can cause neonatal thrombocytopenia, although this condition is not as clinically severe as NAIT. Severe thrombocytopenia ($<50 \times 10^9$/l) occurs in about 10% of neonates with maternal platelet autoantibodies of which about half have platelet counts of $<20 \times 10^9$/l. However, studies have shown that risk of severe haemorrhage, including ICH, is very low in this group of neonates [20].

All neonates with a history of maternal thrombocytopenia should have their platelet counts checked at birth, and if found to be $>150 \times 10^9/l$, no further action is necessary. Thrombocytopenic neonates should have their platelet counts rechecked after 2–3 days, as platelet counts often drop to their lowest levels at this age, after which they tend to resolve spontaneously by the age of 7 days in the majority of neonates. In a small group of neonates, thrombocytopenia may persist up to the age of 12 weeks [20]. In this situation, where the thrombocytopenia is severe (platelet count $<30 \times 10^9/l$ in the first week of life and $<20 \times 10^9/l$ thereafter), treatment with IVIG (400 mg/kg/day for 5 days or 1 g/kg/day for 2 days, total dose 2 g/kg) may be useful [1].

Congenital Infections

A large number of congenitally acquired viral infections can cause fetal and neonatal thrombocytopenia. Although the most commonly identified viral causes of neonatal thrombocytopenia are CMV and rubella, cases due to enteroviruses (Coxsackie A and B and echovirus) can also cause severe, acute thrombocytopenia as can HIV and parvovirus B19. In most cases, thrombocytopenia will be present in combination with other clinical features suggestive of congenital infections, e.g. intracranial calcification, hepatosplenomegaly, jaundice, or 'viral' lymphocytes on the blood film. However, severe thrombocytopenia (platelet count $<50 \times 10^9/l$) that is present in the first days of life and persists for more than the first week is a common feature in congenital infections and may then suggest the diagnosis if other more common clinical features are absent or minimal.

Primary or secondary maternal CMV infection during pregnancy results in intrauterine transmission of CMV in 30–40% of cases, although only 20–25% develop post-natal sequelae, including neonatal thrombocytopenia which may be severe and/or may persist for several months [21]. Prenatal diagnosis of CMV infection should be based on amniocentesis (≥7 weeks after presumed infection). Congenital toxoplasmosis affects 1:2,000–1:3,000 newborns, depending on geographical location and dietary practices. The incidence of thrombocytopenia in affected neonates is approximately 40%. Congenital rubella is now very rare in countries with an active immunization programme but persistent thrombocytopenia is a prominent feature of neonates with congenital rubella syndrome. Congenital parvovirus B19 infection, although more usually associated with fetal anaemia, also not infrequently causes fetal and neonatal thrombocytopenia.

Perinatal Bacterial Infection

Perinatal infection is commonly related to prolonged rupture of membranes and usually presents as early-onset neonatal infection (present by 72 h). Recent studies show that perinatal infection occurs in ~3.5/1,000 births most commonly due to group B *Streptococcus* or *Escherichia coli* [22]. Infections with these organisms are a relatively common cause of stillbirth and also cause serious neonatal morbidity, with thrombocytopenia developing in ~50% of cases. In contrast to late-onset neonatal sepsis, DIC appears to be an important mechanism of thrombocytopenia, probably because of the severity of the sepsis syndrome induced by the causative organisms and the fact that infection has often begun prior to delivery and therefore before effective treatment can be instituted. The blood film shows characteristic prominent left-shifted neutrophils with or without toxic granulation. Worsening thrombocytopenia and neutropenia are poor prognostic signs.

Chromosomal Abnormalities Associated with Neonatal Thrombocytopenia

Fetal thrombocytopenia is common in aneuploidy. Hohlfeld et al. [23] reported frequencies of 86% for trisomy 18, 31% for trisomy 13, 75% for triploidy and 31% for Turner syndrome at fetal diagnosis. Although in this study the frequency of thrombocytopenia in trisomy 21 was only 6%, other studies indicate that thrombocytopenia is common in trisomy 21, particularly by the time of birth [reviewed in 24]. Approximately 10% of neonates with Down syndrome develop a clonal pre-leukaemic condition, transient myeloproliferative disorder (TMD), also known as transient abnormal myelopoiesis, which is characterised by increased peripheral blood myeloblasts, abnormal megakaryocytes and variable thrombocytopenia [24]. In most cases TMD resolves spontaneously, but ~30% of neonates with TMD subsequently develop acute megakaryocytic leukaemia, within the first 5 years of life [24]. Clinically, TMD has a variable neonatal presentation from asymptomatic mild thrombocytopenia to fulminant hepatic fibrosis due to hepatic infiltration with abnormal megakaryocytes and blasts [24]. TMD is due to acquired somatic mutations in the key megakaryocytic transcription factor GATA1.

Inherited Thrombocytopenia

A number of inherited conditions constitute a rare but important group of disorders that present with thrombocytopenia at birth. In the majority of cases, thrombocytopenia occurs as a result of impaired megakaryocytopoiesis due to abnormal stem cell development and some patients may present with other associated congenital anomalies that are useful in guiding clinicians toward appropriate investigations and management. Thrombocytopenia generally presents at birth and persists in the absence of any other symptoms such as sepsis or NEC. Only conditions which commonly present in the neonate are briefly discussed here (table 2).

Table 2. Inherited thrombocytopenias

Name	Pathophysiology	Gene(s)/loci involved
Fanconi anaemia	usually as part of VACTERL syndrome	FANCB in VACTERL syndrome
Thrombocytopenia and absent radius syndrome	unknown; may be in part due to defects in TPO signalling pathway	compound inheritance of a low-frequency noncoding SNP and a rare null allele in RBM8A
Congenital amegakaryocytic thrombocytopenia	abnormal TPO receptor, abnormal megakaryocyte response to TPO	MPL
Bernard Soulier syndrome	qualitative or quantitative defect in platelet glycoprotein GP1b-IX-V complex	GPIbA, GPIbB, GP9
Amegakaryocytic thrombocytopenia with radio-ulnar synostosis (ATRUS)	abnormality in megakaryocyte differentiation due to HOXA11 gene mutation	HOXA11
X-linked thrombocytopenia (XLT)	abnormal megakaryocyte development	GATA1

VACTERL = Vertebral disorders, anal atresia, cardiac anomalies, trachea-oesophageal fistula, oesophageal atresia, renal dysplasia, limb abnormalities; TPO = thrombopoeitin; SNP = single nucleotide polymorphism.

Bernard-Soulier Syndrome

This is an autosomal-recessive disorder characterized by mild to moderate thrombocytopenia, giant platelets, and a prolonged bleeding time. Bernard-Soulier syndrome is due to qualitative or quantitative defects in the GPIb-IX-V complex as a result of mutations in one of the 4 genes encoding the complex. Bleeding is not usually severe in the neonatal period but may occur. Treatment by platelet transfusion is effective but should be reserved for life-threatening haemorrhage since transfused patients may form allo-antibodies against GPIb, GPIX, or GPV.

Congenital Amegakaryocytic Thrombocytopenia

This autosomal-recessive bone marrow failure syndrome typically presents at birth with petechiae and/or other evidence of bleeding, isolated thrombocytopenia and morphologically normal platelets [reviewed in 25]. The platelet count is usually $<20 \times 10^9/l$ at birth and the bone marrow shows normal cellularity with a specific reduction in megakaryocytes. Physical anomalies are present in ~50% of children. Congenital amegakaryocytic thrombocytopenia is caused by mutations in the c-mpl gene in the majority of patients. Approximately 50% of patients subsequently develop childhood aplastic anaemia and there are several reports of myelodysplasia and/or leukaemia developing later in childhood. Treatment in the neonatal period is with platelet transfusion for bleeding episodes.

TAR Syndrome

This syndrome is characterised by bilateral absence of the radii while both thumbs are present, which may be useful in distinguishing this syndrome from Fanconi anaemia. Most babies with TAR syndrome develop thrombocytopenia within the first week of life. The platelet count is usually $<50 \times 10^9/l$ and the white cell count is elevated in >90% of patients, sometimes exceeding $100 \times 10^9/l$ and mimicking congenital leukaemia. There is a high frequency of associated abnormalities particularly cow's milk intolerance, facial dysmorphism and lower limb anomalies. Those infants that survive the first year of life generally do well, since the platelet count spontaneously improves and is usually maintained at low normal levels thereafter. Inheritance of TAR syndrome is complex. Both autosomal recessive and autosomal dominant inheritance patterns occur but neither the molecular basis nor the pathogenesis has yet been identified.

Amegakaryocytic Thrombocytopenia with Radio-Ulnar Synostosis (ATRUS)

Patients with ATRUS present at birth with severe thrombocytopenia, absent bone marrow megakaryocytes and characteristic skeletal abnormalities. In addition to radio-ulnar synostosis, affected infants may have clinodactyly and shallow acetabulae. Two kindreds show that ATRUS is caused by mutations in the HOXA11 gene which disrupt DNA binding.

X-Linked Thrombocytopenia (XLT) due to GATA-1 Mutations

In addition to TMD and acute megakaryocytic leukaemia seen specifically in children with Down syndrome (see above), *GATA1* mutations also cause 2 different forms of inherited thrombocytopenia which differ mainly in their associated red cell abnormalities – XLT with dyserythropoiesis, which may present at birth, and XLT with thalassaemia, which presents towards the end of the first year of life. XLT with dyserythropoiesis presents at birth either with bleeding secondary to severe thrombocytopenia or as fetal hydrops secondary to dyserythropoietic anaemia.

Management of Neonatal Thrombocytopenia

Investigation

We recommend a pragmatic approach in investigating neonatal thrombocytopenia, based on gestational age and age at presentation, to limit over-investigation of mild or self-limiting cases. Figures 1 and 2 show a practical diagnostic algorithm, which can be applied to the diagnosis and investigation of thrombocytopenia in preterm and term neonates respectively. The cause of each episode can usually be determined by a

Table 3. Indications for neonatal platelet transfusion

Platelet count	Clinical indication
$<20 \times 10^9/l$	all neonates
$<30 \times 10^9/l$	neonates of <1,000 g and, <1 week age or with one or more of: clinically unstable (fluctuating BP) previous major bleeding (grade 3–4 IVH) current minor bleeding: petechiae, puncture site oozing, blood-stained ET secretions coagulopathy requiring surgery or exchange transfusion
$<50 \times 10^9/l$	major haemorrhage

BP = Blood pressure; IVH = intraventricular haemorrhage; ET = endotracheal tube. Modified from Gibson et al. [19].

combination of the clinical history, the timing of the onset of thrombocytopenia (tables 1, 2) and the blood count and film. A small proportion of term and preterm neonates (<1%) will have persistent thrombocytopenia and it is these who should have further specialised investigations performed, guided by the presence or not of dysmorphic features or a family history.

Clinical Impact of Neonatal Thrombocytopenia

Most episodes of thrombocytopenia are relatively mild, transient and self-limiting and therefore unlikely to have short-term or long-term consequences. However, for the 5–10% of severe and/or prolonged cases, mortality and morbidity are increased [26]. The most important clinical factors which affect the frequency of major haemorrhage are low birth weight and prematurity. The most common site of major haemorrhage in neonates is intracranial (particularly intraventricular haemorrhage) which is documented in ~5% of all thrombocytopenic neonates, while gastrointestinal haemorrhage occurs in 1–5%, pulmonary haemorrhage in 0.6–5% and haematuria in 1–2% of thrombocytopenic neonates [14]. Low-birth-weight preterm neonates have one of the highest rates of ICH of any age group (up to 25%), and the ICH may be fatal or lead to long-term neurodevelopmental disability [11].

Indications for Platelet Transfusion

Platelet transfusions remain the mainstay of treatment of neonatal thrombocytopenia. Until results of clinical trials to define the role of platelet transfusion in reducing bleeding risk in neonates with severe thrombocytopenia are available, consensus guidelines are used in many countries. Our own practice is based on the British Committee for Standards in Haematology (BCSH) guidelines for platelet transfusion [19], modified to provide two higher thresholds for transfusion for neonates predicted to be at 'high' or 'very high' risk of haemorrhage. 'High risk' neonates are those <28 weeks' gestation, or with a birth weight <1,000 g, are clinically unstable, due for planned surgery, or have minor bleeding or coagulopathy. In these children, we use a transfusion threshold of 30×10^9/l. 'Very high' risk neonates are those with active major haemorrhage and are therefore considered to be at a higher risk of ICH and adverse neurodevelopmental outcome, and we use a threshold of 50×10^9/l in these children (table 3).

Conclusion

Thrombocytopenia is common in neonatal units and has a wide variety of underlying causes. Since the majority of neonates with thrombocytopenia remit spontaneously, with few or no clinical sequelae, it is important to consider the clinical context of the thrombocytopenia to guide rational investigations. The mainstay of treatment of neonatal thrombocytopenia is platelet transfusion using consensus or 'best practice' guidelines which aim to reduce the risk of severe haemorrhage in thrombocytopenic neonates. The outcome of on-going and future studies will be crucial for determining the precise role of platelet transfusion in improving outcome in thrombocytopenic neonates.

References

1 Roberts I, Stanworth S, Murray NA: Thrombocytopenia in the neonate. Blood Reviews 2008;22:173–186.
2 Dreyfus M, Kaplan C, Verdy E, Schlegel N, Durand-Zaleski I, Tchernia G: Immune thrombocytopenia working group. Frequency of immune thrombocytopenia in newborns: a prospective study. Blood 1997;89:4402–4406.
3 Muthukumar P, Venkatesh V, Curley A, Kahan BC, Choo L, Ballard S, Clarke P, Watts MDT, Roberts I, Stanworth S, Platelets Neonatal Transfusion Study Group: Severe thrombocytopenia and patterns of bleeding in neonates: results from a prospective observational study and implications for use of platelet transfusions. Transfus Med 2012;22:338–343.
4 Cremer M, Sola-Visner M, Roll S, Josephson CD, Yilmaz Z, Bührer C, Dame C: Platelet transfusions in neonates: practices in the United States vary significantly from those in Austria, Germany, and Switzerland. Transfusion 2011;51:2634–2641.
5 Ghevaert C, Campbell K, Walton J, Smith GA, Allen D, Williamson LM, Ouwehand WH, Ranasinghe E: Management and outcome of 200 cases of fetomaternal alloimmune thrombocytopenia. Transfusion 2007:47;901–910.
6 Hann IM: Development of blood in the fetus; in Hann IM, Gibson BES, Letsky E (eds): Fetal and Neonatal Haematology, ed 1. London, Bailliere Tindall, 1991, pp 1–28.
7 Wiedemeier SE, Henry E, Sola-Visner M, Christensen RD: Platelet reference ranges for neonates, defined using data from over 47,000 patients in a multi hospital healthcare system. J Perinatol 2009;29: 130–136.
8 Ferrer-Marin F, Liu ZJ, Gutti R, Sola-Visner M: Neonatal thrombocytopenia and megakaryocytopoiesis. Semin Hematol 2010;47:281–288.
9 Liu ZJ, Italiano J Jr, Ferrer-Marin F, Gutti R, Bailey M, Poterjoy B, Rimsza L, Sola-Visner M: Developmental differences in megakaryocytopoiesis are associated with up-regulated TPO signalling through mTOR and elevated GATA-1 levels in neonatal megakaryocytes. Blood 2011;117:4106–4117.
10 Sola-Visner MC, Christensen RD, Hutson AD, Rimsza LM: Megakaryocyte size and concentration in the bone marrow of thrombocytopenic and non-thrombocytopenic neonates. Pediatr Res 2007;61:479–484.
11 Chakravorty S, Roberts I: How I manage neonatal thrombocytopenia. Br J Haematol 2012;156:155–162.

12 Watts TL, Roberts IAG: Haematological abnormalities in the growth-restricted infant. Semin Neonatol 1999;4:41–54.
13 Veldman A, Fischer D, Nold MF, Wong FY: Disseminated intravascular coagulation in term and preterm neonates. Semin Thromb Hemost 2010;36: 419–428.
14 Stanworth SJ, Clarke P, Watts T, Ballard S, Choo L, Morris T, Murphy MF, Roberts I, Platelets and Neonatal Transfusion Study Group: Prospective, observational study of outcomes in neonates with severe thrombocytopenia. Pediatrics 2009;124:e826–e834.
15 Peterson JA, McFarland JG, Curtis BR, Aster RH: Neonatal alloimmune thrombocytopenia: pathogenesis, diagnosis and management. Br J Haematol 2013;161:3–14.
16 Kroll H, Yates J, Santoso S: Immunization against a low-frequency human platelet alloantigen in fetal alloimmune thrombocytopenia is not a single event: characterization by the combined use of reference DNA and novel allele-specific cell lines expressing recombinant antigens. Transfusion 2005;45:353–358.
17 Symington A, Paes B: Fetal and neonatal alloimmune thrombocytopenia: harvesting the evidence to develop a clinical approach to management. Am J Perinatol 2011;28:137–144.
18 Vinograd CA, Bussel JB: Antenatal treatment of fetal alloimmune thrombocytopenia: a current perspective. Haematologica 2010;95:1807–1911.
19 Gibson BE, Todd A, Roberts I, Pamphilon D, Rodeck C, Bolton-Maggs P, Burbin G, Duguid J, Boulton F, Cohen H, Smith N, McClelland DB, Rowley M, Turner G, British Committee for Standards in Haematology Transfusion Task Force: Writing group. Transfusion guidelines for neonates and older children. Br J Haematol 2004;124:433–453.
20 Webert KE, Mittal R, Sigouin C, Heddle NM, Kelton JG: A retrospective 11-year analysis of obstetric patients with idiopathic thrombocytopenic purpura. Blood 2003;102:4306–4311.
21 Liesnard C, Donner C, Brancart F, Gosselin F, Delforge ML, Rodesch F: Prenatal diagnosis of congenital cytomegalovirus infection: prospective study of 237 pregnancies at risk. Obstet Gynecol 2000;95: 881–888.
22 Kuhn P, Dheu C, Bolender C, Chognot D, Keller L, Demil H, Donato L, Langer B, Messer J, Astruc D: Incidence and distribution of pathogens in early-onset neonatal sepsis in the era of antenatal antibiotics. Paediatr Perinat Epidemiol 2010;24:479–487.
23 Hohlfeld P, Forestier F, Kaplan C, Tissot JD, Daffos F: Fetal thrombocytopenia: a retrospective survey of 5,194 fetal blood samplings. Blood 1994;84:1851–1856.
24 Roy A, Roberts I, Norton A, Vyas P: Acute megakaryoblastic leukaemia (AMKL) and transient myeloproliferative disorder (TMD) in Down syndrome: a multi-step model of myeloid leukaemogenesis. Br J Haematol 2009;147:3–12.
25 Geddis AE: Congenital amegakaryocytic thrombocytopenia and thrombocytopenia with absent radii. Hematol Oncol Clin North Am 2010;23:321–331.
26 Garcia MG, Duenas E, Sola M, Hutson AD, Theriaque D, Christensen R: Epidemiologic and outcome studies of patients who received platelet transfusions in the neonatal intensive care unit. J Perinatol 2001; 21:415–420.

Irene Roberts
Centre for Haematology, Hammersmith Campus
Imperial College London
Du Cane Road, London W12 0NN (UK)
E-Mail irene.roberts@imperial.ac.uk

Thomas AE, Halsey C (eds): Controversies in Pediatric and Adolescent Hematology.
Pediatr Adolesc Med. Basel, Karger, 2014, vol 17, pp 16–29 (DOI: 10.1159/000350344)

Paediatric and Adolescent Immune Thrombocytopenia: Prevention of Bleeding versus Burden of Treatment

Nichola Cooper

Hammersmith Hospital, Imperial College, London, UK

Abstract

In the majority of children, immune thrombocytopenia is an acute disease of short duration with mild symptoms. In approximately 20% of children, however, the thrombocytopenia does not resolve. Management of these individuals can be challenging both due to difficulties in diagnosis, which remains one of exclusion, and because of the paucity of clinical trials. Although most children can be managed by careful monitoring, a small proportion of children will suffer from bleeding. Treatment is not aimed to be curative, but is used to prevent life-threatening bleeding such as intracranial haemorrhage, which remains rare. Identifying patients at risk for intracranial haemorrhage is paramount to management. First-line therapy recommendations continue to be steroids or intravenous immunoglobulin. In those who do not go into an early remission, second-line therapies are multiple and include: immunosuppressive agents such as azathioprine and mycophenolate mofetil, splenectomy and increasingly rituximab. For those patients with refractory disease, clinical trials of the new thrombopoietin receptor agonists are promising. Deciding which patients require treatment relates as much to quality-of-life issues, including socializing and fatigue, as to platelet counts and bleeding.

Copyright © 2014 S. Karger AG, Basel

Immune thrombocytopenia (ITP) in children is mostly a short-lived illness, with thrombocytopenia only lasting a few weeks with few, if any, symptoms. In these patients no treatment is usually required. However, a small number of children will develop bleeding, which can be life threatening, and about 20% of children will not go into an immediate remission and will continue to be thrombocytopenic. The wide range of phenotypes in childhood ITP and the lack of a specific diagnostic test make the management of this rare condition challenging. In addition, the infrequent presentation means there are few clinical trials and little evidence-based practice. This is reflected in some of the differences outlined in the 4 published guidelines on ITP (American Society for Hematology (ASH) guidelines 1996 [1], BSH guidelines 2003 [2], Consensus document 2009 [3], ASH 2011 [4]) outlined in table 1.

Definitions

Following a meeting of physicians experienced in the management of ITP, a number of controversial issues were discussed and a consensus reached. The aim of the meeting was to improve the ability to design studies and be able to compare different published studies appropriately. From this consensus, the following terms were defined [5]:

Newly diagnosed ITP: ITP within 3 months of first presentation.

Persistent ITP: ITP lasting between 3 and 12 months.

Chronic ITP: ITP lasting more than 12 months.

Refractory ITP: ITP refractory to standard treatment.

Response criteria to treatment were also defined. These standards have helped in comparison of different treatment types, and in addition, aim to streamline future studies better.

Diagnosis of Immune Thrombocytopenia

The diagnosis of ITP remains one of exclusion. Thrombocytopenia can be caused by a number of pathologies and ITP itself is associated with many other immune mediated conditions. Taking a careful history is important and can establish most secondary causes, such as other platelet disorders (suggested by bleeding out of proportion to the platelet count or a family history of thrombocytopenia) and other autoimmune disorders such as systemic lupus erythematosus where a history of rash, mouth ulcers or hair loss may be elicited. Investigations to exclude other causes can be tailored to the history and examination findings. Other causes of an isolated thrombocytopenia in children are shown in table 2. Antiplatelet antibodies are currently thought not to be sensitive or specific enough for diagnosis and are not recommended [3, 4].

Whether a bone marrow examination should be performed remains contentious. In those who have no other significant abnormalities, such as other cytopenias, organomegaly or abnormalities on blood film examination, a bone marrow examination is not required, especially if no treatment is indicated. Although the 2003 guidelines recommend bone marrow examination if treatment with steroids is likely in case these may mask acute leukaemia [2], in patients who have a typical history, a normal phys-

Table 1. Comparison of consensus and guidelines

	International consensus document, 2009 [3]	ASH evidence-based practice guidelines, 2011 [4]
Diagnosis	Igs in basic evaluation, ANA recommended in those with persistent disease (>3 months)	insufficient evidence to support routine use of APAs, ANA, TPO levels, platelet parameters
Bone marrow	only recommended when other abnormalities are present, including unexplained enlarged spleen, bone pain, abnormal FBC or blood film, in those who do not respond to first-line therapies	only if other abnormalities in history, physical examination, FBC or film
Factors affecting whether to treat	platelet count, activity profile, psychosocial issues	assessment of impact on daily life. How is the patient coping psychologically with having a low platelet count?
Steroids	short course recommended	short course recommended
Rituximab	has been used with success in children with chronic refractory ITP; well tolerated	may be considered in children who have significant ongoing bleeding and/or have a need for improved quality of life despite conventional treatment; may also be considered as an alternative to splenectomy
Splenectomy	splenectomy rarely recommended. Post splenectomy sepsis is up to 3% in children	chronic or persistent ITP with significant or persistent bleeding and lack of response, or intolerance to other therapies. Should be delayed for at least 12 months, unless severe disease unresponsive to other measures, or due to quality of life considerations
Immuno-supression	experience is limited and therefore no recommendation can be made	multiple agents have been reported; but data for any specific agent remain insufficient for specific recommendations
High-dose dexamethasone		may be considered in children or adolescents who have significant ongoing bleeding and/or have a need for improved quality of life despite conventional treatment; may also be considered as an alternative to splenectomy
TPORs	insufficient evidence at time of publication; may be of value both for chronic disease and those not responsive to first-line therapies, if safety continues	insufficient evidence at time of publication

Igs = Immunoglobulins; ANA = antinuclear antibodies; APA = anti-platelet antibodies; TPO = thrombopoietin; FBC = full blood count; TPOR = thrombopoietin receptor agonists.

Table 2. Alternative causes of thrombocytopenia

Pseudothrombocytopenia (platelet clumping)	
	Laboratory artefact
	Type 2B von Willebrand disease
Congenital thrombocytopenias	
Small platelets (MPV <7 fl)	
	Wiskott-Aldrich syndrome
	X-linked thrombocytopenia
Normal sized platelets (MPV 7–11 fl)	
	CAMT
	TAR syndrome, thrombocytopenia and radial synostosis
	Familial platelet disorder/acute myeloid leukemia
Large/giant platelets (MPV >11 fl)	
	MYH9-related thrombocytopenia
	Bernard-Soulier syndrome
	Gray platelet syndrome
	Velocardiofacial/DiGeorge syndrome
	Paris-Trousseau thrombocytopenia/Jacobsen syndrome
Other	
	Splenomegaly
	Storage disorders, such as Gaucher disease

MPV = Mean platelet volume; CAMT = congenital amegakaryocytic thrombocytopenia; TAR = thrombocytopenia and absent radius syndrome.

ical examination and a normal blood smear, apart from thrombocytopenia, the procedure can be avoided as acute leukaemia is very unlikely; subsequent reviews reflect this by not recommending routine bone marrow examination [3, 4]. In those with an atypical presentation, either with other worrying clinical signs, or other features on the blood count or blood film, all reviews recommend a bone marrow examination. Similarly, in patients who do not respond to standard medications a bone marrow examination should also be considered [3, 4].

Pathogenesis of Immune Thrombocytopenia

Studies in the 1950s first identified a plasma-derived factor initiating thrombocytopenia, when medical students who were injected with plasma from patients with ITP developed a profound thrombocytopenia [6]. Subsequent studies revolved around the discovery of an anti-platelet antibody. Although apparently causative in at least some patients, identification of the anti-platelet antibody, and subsequent utilization for both diagnosis and assessment of treatment responses has been elusive. Furthermore, it has never been clear whether the anti-platelet antibody is the prime pathological event, or whether the T cells, which co-ordinate the immune system are more likely to be where the problem arises. Evaluation of the T cell compartment in ITP reveals many abnormalities. These include skewing towards Th1 phenotype [7], with a reduction in Th2 cells [8], a reduction in the quantity and functional ability of regulatory T cells [9] and the ability of cytotoxic T cells to destroy platelets directly [10]. Other controlling factors including regulatory B cells and monocytes are also under investigation. These defects in the immune system also appear to affect the ability of megakaryocytes to produce platelets with decreased megakaryocyte proliferation in the presence of ITP plasma [11]. While the abnormalities in the immune system appear widespread, a causative agent remains unknown. Associations with infectious agents, including bacteria *(Helicobacter pylori)* and viruses (hepatitis B, hepatitis C and human immunodeficiency virus) in adults suggest that responses to infections may be the precipitating cause, although this remains unclear [12].

Examination of the pathogenesis of paediatric ITP is more limited. The clinical presentation and progression of ITP in children appears different from adults. Although there is likely to be overlap with adult disease, this remains relatively unexplored. Exploration of genetic factors specific for susceptibility to ITP and evaluation of apoptosis of platelets in children with ITP are potential avenues of investigation.

Vaccination and Immune Thrombocytopenia

Transient thrombocytopenia has been reported after infections, including measles and varicella. It has also been reported after vaccinations, potentially up to 1 in 40,000 cases of MMR vaccination [13]. The episodes are usually transient and mild. The actual incidence is difficult to ascertain, but is unlikely to be more frequent or more severe than the thrombocytopenia following the illnesses themselves. Whether using multiple vaccinations at the same time increases the risk of thrombocytopenia will be even more difficult to establish given the low frequency of the episodes. For example, one study analysed data from 5 managed care organisations from 2000 to 2009. This included a cohort of 1.8 million children of ages 6 weeks to 17 years. Using diagnostic codes, those developing ITP were identified and platelet counts were taken and verified by chart review. Incidence ratios were calculated to compare the risk of ITP 1–42 days after vaccination. Overall, there were only 197 confirmed cases of ITP. There was an increased risk after MMR vaccination, as has been reported previously, but no other associations could be established because of the small numbers of patients [14].

Management

The majority of children with ITP will not suffer bleeding symptoms, despite having low platelet counts. Treatment is aimed at preventing significant haemorrhage, which remains rare.

Successive guidelines have shown a decreasing trend to advise treatment for children with uncomplicated ITP. Interestingly, more emphasis is also put on psychological effects, with the ASH guideline clearly stating that the patient should be evaluated for the psychological effect of a low platelet count [4]. Assessment of psychosocial issues and level of activity is also discussed in the consensus document [3]. The consensus document also discusses a modified bleeding/quality-of-life score ranging from 1, with minor bleeding and few petechiae to grade 4 with mucosal bleeding or suspected internal haemorrhage. For patients with either no symptoms or only cutaneous symptoms (grade 1 or 2), it is suggested that only selected children need treatment; intervention is only recommended with grade 3 (mucosal bleeding and troublesome lifestyle) and grade 4 symptoms.

In the UK, there is an increasing trend not to treat children with ITP. A recent paper analysing results from the UK registry data shows decreasing treatment rates of from 61% in 1995 to 16% in 2011 [15]. This summary also showed there was no impact on the incidence of intracranial haemorrhage.

However, the impact of ITP is not only due to the risk of significant bleeding, as small bleeds may have an undocumented effect, and concern and anxiety over low platelet counts and perceived risks also have a significant effect on the children's and parents' lives.

Quality of Life and Fatigue

Increasingly, quality of life-related questionnaires are being used to assess patients with ITP. Health-related quality of life (HRQoL) scores in adults with ITP equate to other chronic disorders and patients remain anxious about their disease. Treatments can improve HRQoL, although it is not clear whether this is a psychological effect of having a 'normal' platelet count or a physiological effect of platelets and/or the correction of the immune imbalance.

The kids ITP tools score was specifically designed to assess children with ITP together with their parents [16]. Interestingly, in one study, parents performed poorly, with low scores that increased when their children were treated with romiplostim. There was no significant effect (although there was a trend to improvement) on the children's scores [17].

In another assessment, a questionnaire-based survey was distributed through the ITP support organization to both adults and children with primary ITP in the United Kingdom: 94 children responded. Children were more likely than adults to experience frustration over activity restrictions (23.3 vs. 9.5%, respectively; $p < 0.001$). Notably, 12.5% of all patients with primary ITP (adults and children) reported 'always' or 'often' missing work or school due to fatigue. These absences were not significantly associated with disease severity ($p = 0.301$) [18].

Fatigue has also become increasingly recognized in patients with ITP. Patients and parents frequently report increased fatigue and irritability when platelets are low. In a retrospective analysis of the notes of 27 children with ITP, fatigue was reported in 6 children (22%). Fatigue did not appear to be related to treatments, to other medical problems or occurrence of anaemia as these patients were excluded from analysis. Although only a retrospective analysis of notes, this is a reasonable percentage of patients, and may be higher with further evaluation [19].

Appropriate analysis of the degree of fatigue is important. While overtreatment is inappropriate, restricting children in both physical and mental activities due to fatigue is also of concern, and may be a reason to treat.

Lifestyle Issues

In patients who are not receiving treatment, lifestyle issues should be discussed, such as avoidance of high-risk sports. In addition, it must be remembered to advise patients/parents not to use antiplatelet drugs. Tranexamic acid can be a very useful treatment for mild bleeding symptoms and is especially useful for menstrual bleeding in older girls. In all patients, whether on observation or active treatment, easy access to expert evaluation is paramount. Clear advice on when children need to be assessed following falls or when active bleeding is evident must be given.

Medical Therapy

In patients who do require therapy, a number of agents can be used, most of which remain unlicensed. The aim of treatment is to induce a rapid increase in the platelet count to a safe haemostatic level, with the least toxicity.

First-Line Treatment

First-line therapy recommendations in children with bleeding include: a short course of oral prednisolone 3–4 mg/kg/day for 4 days (without subsequent tapering) or intravenous immunoglobulin (IVIG) 0.8 g/kg as a single dose. If platelet counts remain low at 24 h, a second dose of IVIG may be given [3, 4]. The majority of children will respond to either of these measures. There are no guidelines for the maximum dose of steroids for an older child. This is an important area which needs addressing. A recent informal poll of physicians in the UK with an interest in ITP showed a wide range of upper limit doses. Further evaluation of the registry data may allow us to better understand both responses to higher doses and toleration of side effects.

Intravenous anti-D has also been used in Rh-positive children with acute ITP and is recommended as the first-line therapy in those with contraindications for steroids in both the consensus document and guidelines [3, 4]. However, it was withdrawn from the EU market in 2010 and there is a black box warning regarding the use of intravenous anti-D in patients with ITP due to the rare complication of severe intravascular haemolysis and disseminated intravascular coagulation, resulting in some deaths. This is a rare and unpredictable complication and appears to be more common in subjects over 60 years of age, those with malignant conditions such as lymphoma, and patients with active viral infections such as Epstein-Barr virus. In the USA, it is now recommended only for patients with severe ITP refractory to other treatments. Exclusion criteria include: patients with leukaemia, lymphoma, EBV or hepatitis C infections, in those older than 65 years, and those with conditions which make them more likely to develop haemolysis (Evan's syndrome, systemic lupus erythematosus, antiphospholipid syndrome). In addition, it is recommended that patients remain under observation for 8 h, which abrogates some of the advantages of anti-D (i.e. its short infusion time) [20].

Management of Chronic Immune Thrombocytopenia

Management of those children who do not go into immediate remission remains challenging. There are no curative treatments apart from possibly splenectomy and treatment revolves around finding treatments with the least toxicity to provide a platelet count sufficient to avoid bleeding. However, finding a 'safe' platelet count has been difficult to establish. As reflected in the consensus and guideline documents, a platelet count above 30×10^9/l is generally considered safe, but may be higher than necessary for most patients.

Long-term use of corticosteroids should be avoided because of predictable toxicities including weight gain, mood disturbances, osteopenia, and, in rare cases, osteonecrosis, hypertension and disorders of glucose regulation. Furthermore, in assessments of impact on lifestyles, the side effects of steroids become one of the biggest burdens, both in children and in family members.

Rituximab

Rituximab therapy is not licensed for use in ITP in adults or children but is increasingly being used in children who continue to suffer from bleeding symptoms. A recent review of the use in children reports similar efficacy to adult ITP, although typically responses appear of shorter duration [21]. An increased proportion of children develop serum infusion reaction type effects. Long-term adverse effects and safety are yet to be established. Hypogammaglobulinaemia does occur in some patients with repeated use [22]. It is not currently clear which patients are more susceptible; however, this has to be considered in children, in whom the immune system is immature and in whom the autoimmunity may reflect other abnormalities of the immune system. An abstract at the American Society of Haematology 2012 showed evidence of poor responses to vaccinations, including pneumovax, in adults who received rituximab. This has also been demonstrated in patients with lymphoma treated with rituximab [23]. Vaccination is now recommended before treatment. Progressive multifocal leukoencephalopathy remains extremely rare although it has occurred in adults with ITP receiving rituximab [24]. Patients who are positive for hepatitis B serology should not be given rituximab. The dose has also not been established. Although low doses, 100 mg weekly for 4 weeks have been used with success in adults [25], it is not certain whether duration of effect will be the same as the standard dose (375 mg/m^2) used in patients with lymphoma, or 1 g BD used in rheumatoid arthritis. In adults, using rituximab together with dexamethasone may induce more and longer remissions (this is currently under evaluation). While there is clear benefit for children who respond and do not need treatment for up to a year (or more in those who do not relapse), this has to be balanced by the potential risk of repeated depletion of B cells. The overall benefit:risk balance is not known.

Azathioprine and Mycophenolate Mofetil

Immunosuppressive agents, including azathioprine and mycophenolate mofetil can be very useful in adults and children with autoimmune disorders. Generally, they are well tolerated. There is anxiety around their long-term use, with concerns about increased risks of malignancy. However, these agents, particularly azathioprine, have been used in many conditions with little toxicity. It can be a very useful steroid-sparing agent, although few studies are reported on its use in ITP. Both the consensus and guidelines documents do not feel there is significant evidence to recommend their use in paediatric ITP [3, 4].

Splenectomy

Splenectomy remains the only treatment that offers the potential of cure. In children with chronic ITP, response rates are around 70% [summarized in ref. 26].

However, there is considerable difference in opinions regarding splenectomy; this is reflected in the guidelines for management of ITP. Most agree that splenectomy should be reserved for children in whom platelets remain low for more than 12 months and in whom either the low platelet or other treatments are significantly interfering with daily activity or constituting a significant risk of morbidity or mortality [1–4].

However, many patients are reluctant to undergo surgery, especially given the risk of not responding, or of relapse. Splenic destruction scans appear to be helpful [27].

Furthermore, the long-term consequences of splenectomy are not well known. Potential increased risks of thrombosis and pulmonary hypertension are beginning to be evaluated. This needs to be considered alongside the long-term side effects of other therapies, and the long-term effects of persistent thrombocytopenia.

Vaccinations and Antibiotic Prophylaxis

Before elective splenectomy children should be fully immunized against encapsulated bacteria (*Streptococcus pneumoniae*, *Haemophilus influenzae* type b, and *Neisseria meningitidis*).

The need for antibiotic prophylaxis with penicillin, or an equivalent antibiotic in patients who are allergic to penicillin, following splenectomy also continues to be debated. Most reports recommend that prophylaxis with penicillin is given to all children <5 years of age with asplenia and for 2 years after splenectomy in older children. In the UK life-long antibiotic prophylaxis is recommended. Travel abroad needs to be carefully planned with additional measures taken when travelling to remote areas where medical attention cannot easily be given or areas endemic for malaria or meningitis. For example, vaccination with a meningococcal A, C, W135 and Y conjugate vaccine such as Menveo is recommended.

Thrombopoietin Agonists

Thrombopoietin (TPO) agonists are novel agents, specifically designed to increase the platelet count. Two agents are currently licensed for use in adults, with other agents in development. Both agents work through the TPO receptor (previously called the MPL receptor) although with different modes of action.

Romiplostim (AMG 53, Nplate, Amgen) is a recombinant protein classified as a peptibody. It is comprised of two IgG Fc domains, which cause it to be recycled, extending its half-life, coupled with four copies of a TPO mimetic peptide. It activates the TPO receptor through its TPO-binding site. It is given as a subcutaneous injection once a week. In placebo-controlled studies in adults, it showed greater response rates and reduction in rescue medications in treatment compared with non-treatment arms, in both splenectomised and non-splenectomised patients. In a long-term extension study, 87% of patients had a platelet response, with 78% of patients maintaining counts more than 50×10^9/l for more than 10 weeks [28].

In children, the results from two randomized controlled studies have been published. The largest describes 15/17 children (88%) with a response to romiplostim (platelet count $\geq 50 \times 10^9$/l) compared to none of the patients receiving placebo. The median weekly dose was higher in children (5 μg/kg). There were no treatment-related serious adverse events. The most commonly reported adverse events in children, as in adults, were headache and epistaxis [29]. In a second study, 10/12 (83.3%) responded to romiplostim, again with no serious adverse events [30].

Eltrombopag (SB-497115 GSK) is an oral agent taken once a day. It is a small molecule which activates the TPO receptor at the transmembrane domain, and not at the TPO binding site. It has been shown to have a similar efficacy to romiplostim, although no comparative studies have been performed.

In RAISE, a randomized controlled study comparing etlrombopag to placebo, patients receiving eltrombopag had greater odds of achieving the primary outcome of a platelet count between $50 \times 10^9/l$ and $400 \times 10^9/l$ during the 6-month treatment period than placebo (OR 8.2, 99% CI 3.6, 18.7). In patients receiving eltrombopag, 50/83 (60%) of non-splenectomised patients and 18/49 (37%) of splenectomised patients achieved counts $>50 \times 10^9/l$. The median duration of response was 10.9 weeks for eltrombopag compared with 0 weeks for placebo. Patients receiving eltrombopag required less rescue medication and had lower odds of bleeding events [31]. A 3-year extension study in 299 patients treated with eltrombopag shows no new safety data with 80–88% of patients achieving a platelet count $>50 \times 10^9/l$ at least once [32]. Results from studies in children will shortly be available.

The safety and tolerability in adults for both agents has been good, with little difference between the placebo and treatment arms.

Specific Side Effects Include

1 Thromboembolic events appeared higher than expected (around 5%) in both studies and on both the placebo and the treatment arms. There was no statistically significant difference between placebo and treatment arms, suggesting the thrombotic risk may relate to ITP itself. This is likely to be less of an issue in paediatrics, where thromboembolic risks events are rare.
2 Reticulin deposition increases in a small number of patients and has resulted in a leukoerythroblastic blood picture with cytopenias. This appears to be reversible on stopping treatment and has had no long-term effects so far, although is subject to further examination.
3 Increased liver function tests are seen in some patients treated with eltrombopag. This also appears reversible and no patient has gone on to develop irreversible liver disease.
4 Rebound thrombocytopenia occurs if the agents are stopped abruptly.
5 Fluctuating platelet counts can be difficult to manage, and may require dual ITP therapy with low dose steroids, or other T cell therapy such as mycophenolate mofetil or cyclosporine (anecdotal reports and case reports only).

Some investigative studies suggest that there may be an additional immune tolerance effect with TPO agents [9], and a proportion of patients are able to come off treatment altogether (reported in both ASH and European Hematology Association

(EHA) abstracts). There is a theoretical concern about the long-term stimulation of the bone marrow, particularly in children. Long-term safety studies are required to show whether this is a real issue.

Conclusion

The first stage in the management of childhood ITP relates to making the correct diagnosis. This involves standard history taking, and relies on the exclusion of other causes, in particular other thrombocytopenic conditions or immunologic disorders.

There has been much change and progress in the management of children with ITP. First it is clear that few children need treatment. Second if treatment is required, then there are a number of new steroid-sparing agents including rituximab and the thrombopoietic agents, which show promise with low side effects, at least in the short term. Understanding when to use these agents and further evaluation of their long-term effects is vital in patient care. Furthermore, better education of what constitutes a risk, e.g. when should parents take children to A and E for assessment if they are not being treated, is important.

Bleeding is not the only consideration in managing children with ITP. HRQoL surveys suggest that children are missing school because of thrombocytopenia and that children are frustrated about the recommendations for decreased activity and socialising. Finally, the anxiety created around not treating and the potential risks of bleeding are likely to impact on the parent-child relationship and may influence the development into young adults.

Appropriately designed controlled studies, which include HRQoL scores and long-term follow-up are required in order to evaluate whether treating or not treating children with ITP has an impact on life. In addition, identifying other risk factors for bleeding and better understanding of the toxicities of treatment is needed. Managing ITP is currently managing a balance of risks, many of which are not yet fully understood.

References

1 George JN, Woolf SH, Raskob GE, Wasser JS, Aledort LM, Ballem PJ, Blanchette VS, Bussel JB, Cines DB, Kelton JG, Lichtin AE, McMillan R, Okerbloom JA, Regan DH, Warrier I: Idiopathic thrombocytopenic purpura: a practice guideline developed by explicit methods for the American Society of Hematology. Blood 1996;88:3–40.

2 British Committee for Standards in Haematology General Haematology Task Force: Guidelines for the investigation and management of idiopathic thrombocytopenic purpura in adults, children and in pregnancy. Br J Haematol 2003;120:574–596.

3 Provan D, Stasi R, Newland AC, Blanchette VS, Bolton-Maggs P, Bussel JB, Chong BH, Cines DB, Gernsheimer TB, Godeau B, Grainger J, Greer I, Hunt BJ, Imbach PA, Lyons G, McMillan R, Rodeghiero F, Sanz MA, Tarantino M, Watson S, Young J, Kuter DJ: International consensus report on the investigation and management of primary immune thrombocytopenia. Blood 2010;115:168–186.

4 Neunert C, Lim W, Crowther M, Cohen A, Solberg L Jr, Crowther MA; American Society of Hematology: The American Society of Hematology 2011 evidence-based practice guideline for immune thrombocytopenia. Blood 2011;117:4190–4207.

5 Rodeghiero F, Stasi R, Gernsheimer T, Michel M, Provan D, Arnold DM, Bussel JB, Cines DB, Chong BH, Cooper N, Godeau B, Lechner K, Mazzucconi MG, McMillan R, Sanz MA, Imbach P, Blanchette V, Kühne T, Ruggeri M, George JN: Standardization of terminology, definitions and outcome criteria in immune thrombocytopenic purpura of adults and children: report from an international working group. Blood 2009;113:2386–2393.

6 Harrington WJ, Minnich V, Hollingsworth JW, Moore CV: Demonstration of a thrombocytopenic factor in the blood of patients with thrombocytopenic purpura. J Lab Clin Med 1951;38:1–10.

7 Semple JW, Milev Y, Cosgrave D, et al: Differences in serum cytokine levels in acute and chronic autoimmune thrombocytopenic purpura: relationship to platelet phenotype and antiplatelet T-cell reactivity. Blood 1996;87:4245–4254.

8 Stasi R, Del Poeta G, Stipa E, et al: Response to B-cell depleting therapy with rituximab reverts the abnormalities of T-cell subsets in patients with idiopathic thrombocytopenic purpura. Blood 2007;110:2924–2930.

9 Bao W, Bussel JB, Heck S, He W, Karpoff M, Boulad N, Yazdanbakhsh K: Improved regulatory T-cell activity in patients with chronic immune thrombocytopenia treated with thrombopoietic agents. Blood 2010;116:4639–4645.

10 Olsson B, Andersson PO, Jernas M, et al: T-cell-mediated cytotoxicity toward platelets in chronic idiopathic thrombocytopenic purpura. Nat Med 2003;9: 1123–1124.

11 McMillan R, Wang L, Tomer A, Nichol J, Pistillo J: Suppression of in vitro megakaryocyte production by antiplatelet autoantibodies from adult patients with chronic ITP. Blood 2004;103:1364–1369.

12 Cines DB, Bussel JB, Liebman HA, Luning Prak ET: The ITP syndrome: pathogenic and clinical diversity. Blood 2009;113:6511–6521.

13 Mantadakis E, Farmaki E, Buchanan GR: Thrombocytopenic purpura after measles-mumps-rubella vaccination: a systematic review of the literature and guidance for management. J Pediatr 2010;156:623–628.

14 O'Leary ST, Glanz JM, McClure DL, Akhtar A, Daley MF, Nakasato C, Baxter R, Davis RL, Izurieta HS, Lieu TA, Ball R: The risk of immune thrombocytopenic purpura after vaccination in children and adolescents. Pediatrics 2012;129:248–255.

15 Grainger JD, Rees JL, Reeves M, Bolton-Maggs PH: Changing trends in the UK management of childhood ITP. Arch Dis Child 2012;97:8–11.

16 Klaassen RJ, Blanchette VS, Barnard D, Wakefield CD, Curtis C, Bradley CS, Neufeld EJ, Buchanan GR, Silva MP, Chan AK, Young NL: Validity, reliability, and responsiveness of a new measure of health-related quality of life in children with immune thrombocytopenic purpura: the Kids' ITP Tools. J Pediatr 2007;150:510–515.

17 Klaassen RJ, Mathias SD, Buchanan G, Bussel J, Deuson R, Young NL, Collier A, Bomgaars L, Blanchette V: Pilot study of the effect of romiplostim on child health-related quality of life (HRQoL) and parental burden in immune thrombocytopenia (ITP). Pediatr Blood Cancer 2012;58:395–398.

18 Sarpatwari A, Watson S, Erqou S, Anderson H, Grainger J, Higgins JP, Newland AC: Health-related lifestyle in adults and children with primary immune thrombocytopenia (ITP). Br J Haematol 2010;151: 189–191.

19 Blatt J, Weston B, Gold S: Fatigue as marker of thrombocytopenia in childhood idiopathic thrombocytopenic purpura. Pediatr Hematol Oncol 2010; 27:65–67.

20 http://www.mhra.gov.uk/Safetyinformation/Safetywarningsalertsandrecalls/Safetywarningsandmessagesformedicines/Monthlylistsofinformationforhealthcareprofessionalsonthesafetyofmedicines/CON057078.

21 Cooper N, Bussel JB: The long-term impact of rituximab for childhood immune thrombocytopenia. Curr Rheumatol Rep 2010;12:94–100.

22 Cooper N, Davies EG, Thrasher AJ: Repeated courses of rituximab for autoimmune cytopenias may precipitate profound hypogammaglobulinaemia requiring replacement intravenous immunoglobulin. Br J Haematol 2009;146:120–122.

23 Yri OE, Torfoss D, Hungnes O, Tierens A, Waalen K, Nordøy T, Dudman S, Kilander A, Wader KF, Ostenstad B, Ekanger R, Meyer P, Kolstad A: Rituximab blocks protective serologic response to influenza A (H1N1) 2009 vaccination in lymphoma patients during or within 6 months after treatment. Blood 2011; 118:6769–6771.

24 Carson KR, Evens AM, Richey EA, Habermann TM, Focosi D, Seymour JF, Laubach J, Bawn SD, Gordon LI, Winter JN, Furman RR, Vose JM, Zelenetz AD, Mamtani R, Raisch DW, Dorshimer GW, Rosen ST, Muro K, Gottardi-Littell NR, Talley RL, Sartor O, Green D, Major EO, Bennett CL: Progressive multifocal leukoencephalopathy after rituximab therapy in HIV-negative patients: a report of 57 cases from the Research on Adverse Drug Events and Reports project. Blood 2009;113:4834–4840.

25 Provan D, Butler T, Evangelista ML, Amadori S, Newland AC, Stasi R: Activity and safety profile of low-dose rituximab for the treatment of autoimmune cytopenias in adults. Haematologica 2007;92: 1695–1698.

26 Breakey VR, Blanchette VS: Childhood immune thrombocytopenia: a changing therapeutic landscape. Semin Thromb Hemost 2011;37:745–755.
27 Sarpatwari A, Provan D, Erqou S, Sobnack R, David Tai FW, Newland AC: Autologous 111 In-labelled platelet sequestration studies in patients with primary immune thrombocytopenia (ITP) prior to splenectomy: a report from the United Kingdom ITP Registry. Br J Haematol 2010;151:477–487.
28 Bussel JB, Kuter DJ, Pullarkat V, Lyons RM, Guo M, Nichol JL: Safety and efficacy of long-term treatment with romiplostim in thrombocytopenic patients with chronic ITP. Blood 2009;113:2161–2171.
29 Bussel JB, Buchanan GR, Nugent DJ, Gnarra DJ, Bomgaars LR, Blanchette VS, Wang YM, Nie K, Jun S: A randomized, double-blind study of romiplostim to determine its safety and efficacy in children with immune thrombocytopenia. Blood 2011;118:28–36.
30 Elalfy MS, Abdelmaksoud AA, Eltonbary KY: Romiplostim in children with chronic refractory ITP: randomized placebo controlled study. Ann Hematol 2011;90:1341–1344.
31 Cheng G, Saleh MN, Marcher C, Vasey S, Mayer B, Aivado M, Arning M, Stone NL, Bussel JB: Eltrombopag for management of chronic immune thrombocytopenia (RAISE): a 6-month, randomised, phase 3 study. Lancet 2011;377:393–402.
32 Saleh MN, Bussel JB, Cheng G, Meyer O, Bailey CK, Arning M, Brainsky A; on behalf of the EXTEND Study Group: Safety and efficacy of eltrombopag for treatment of chronic immune thrombocytopenia: results of the long-term, open-label EXTEND study. Blood 2013;121:537–545.

Nichola Cooper
Hammersmith Hospital, Imperial College
Du Cane Road, London W12 0HS (UK)
E-Mail n.cooper@imperial.ac.uk

Thomas AE, Halsey C (eds): Controversies in Pediatric and Adolescent Hematology.
Pediatr Adolesc Med. Basel, Karger, 2014, vol 17, pp 30–41 (DOI: 10.1159/000350345)

Thrombosis in Paediatrics: Genetic versus Environmental Risk Factors and Implications for Management

Paul Monagle

Department of Paediatrics, University of Melbourne, Royal Children's Hospital, Melbourne, Vic., Australia

Abstract

Virchow, the famous German pathologist, described the three critical factors for the development of thrombosis as being disturbances in blood flow, abnormalities in the blood vessel wall, and disturbances in the blood constituents that led to hypercoagulability. Over 150 years later, this triad remains perhaps the most useful way to think about risk factors for thrombosis, and to consider the relative contributions of genetic versus environmental factors contributing to thrombosis. As will be demonstrated throughout this chapter, environmental risk factors seem far more important to the aetiology, presentation, and management of thrombosis in children than do genetic factors. One cannot conclude that genetic factors play no role; however, the available evidence supports that in a multi-hit causation model, the major causative factors for thrombosis in children are acquired clinical, pathological and iatrogenic factors. Thus, in managing thrombosis in children, it is the amelioration of these factors that are the most important. However, there remains much to be learnt about the interaction of the coagulation system in children and the pathogenesis of thrombosis.

Copyright © 2014 S. Karger AG, Basel

In 1856, Rudolph Virchow, the famous German pathologist, described a triad of factors that he believed led to the formation of venous thrombosis. The three critical factors were disturbances in blood flow, abnormalities in the blood vessel wall, and disturbances in the blood constituents that led to hypercoagulability. Over 150 years later, this triad remains perhaps the most useful way to think about risk factors for thrombosis. The pathogenesis of thrombosis is not simple, and it is likely that multiple abnormalities combine to create pathological thrombosis. There are some aetiological factors which have their impact through multiple components of Virchow's triad. For example, central venous access devices (CVADs) undoubtedly cause local obstruction to blood flow, but also provide an artificial surface within the blood vessel, and alter the propensity of the native blood vessel wall to trigger thrombosis through damage at the insertion site. Coexistent infection may release inflammatory mediators which impact on the blood constituents. However, the questions often asked are: What is the balance of significance between genetic and environmental risk factors? How hard should the clinician look for one, when there is already evidence of the other? What impact does the presence or absence of this balance of risk factors have on patient management?

This chapter will focus on venous thromboembolism, describing the epidemiology of thrombosis in children, discussing risk factors in the context of Virchow's triad, before arguing that in most cases of childhood thrombosis, environmental risk factors are by far the most dominant, and it is the ongoing presence or absence of these factors that should impact on management decisions.

Epidemiology of Thrombosis in Neonates and Children

There would appear little doubt that the epidemiology of childhood thrombosis is changing over time (table 1). This likely relates to increased clinical suspicion, and improved imaging and diagnostic strategies; however, the consensus amongst experts is that the true rate of thrombosis is increasing as children survive more and more complex and severe primary disorders. The concept that thrombosis is a disease of tertiary paediatric care, by definition points towards environmental factors as being the primary causation in paediatric thrombosis.

Aetiology of Venous Thrombosis in Neonates and Children

Abnormalities of Blood Flow

Abnormalities in blood flow may be local or systemic. While local genetic or congenital abnormalities in blood flow (vascular anomalies) can be associated with thrombosis, the overwhelming majority of local interruptions to flow are iatrogenic, with an additional significant proportion being disease related. Table 2 describes the common genetic/congenital versus environmental disturbances in local blood flow that have been described as causing thrombosis in children. Systemic abnormalities to blood flow, such as hypotension, dehydration, polycythaemia or hyperviscosity often contribute to thrombosis as secondary insults acting in conjunction with local problems to precipitate a thrombotic event.

The single most frequently implicated interruption to local blood flow in the aetiology of thrombosis in children is the presence of CVADs. Arguably, CVADs cause thrombosis through interruption of the blood vessel wall at the insertion site, and via producing an abnormal blood vessel wall (the intraluminal surface of the catheter). The importance of the side (left or right) of jugular CVAD placement in the frequency of associated

Table 1. The reported incidence of thrombosis in children

Author	Year	Time interval	Methodology	Age group	Thrombosis type	Hospital incidence	Population incidence
Andrew et al. [16]	1994	2.5 years (1990–1992)	Canadian registry	1 month to 18 years	venous/ PE	5.3/10,000 admissions	0.07/10,000
Van Ommen et al. [17]	2001	2 years (1997–1998)	Dutch registry	0–18 years	venous		0.14/10,000
Gibson et al. [18]	2004	2 years (2001–2003)	BPSU	1 month to 16 years	venous and arterial		0.07/10,000
Newall et al. [19]	2006	4 years (1999–2003)	Single centre series	1 day to 17 years and 7 months	venous	8.0/10,000	
Schmidt and Andrew [20]	1995	3.5 years (1989–1993)	Canadian and International registry	neonates (1 month to 44 weeks)	venous and arterial	24/10,000	
Nowak Gottl et al. [21]	1997	2 years (1992–1994)	German national survey	neonates, up to 4 weeks age	venous and arterial		0.51/10,000
Wright and Watts [22]	2011	3 years (2006–2008)	single centre retro-spective analysis	patients discharged from tertiary paediatric hospital	venous	21.9/10,000	
Setty et al. [23]	2012	1 year 2006	USA inpatient database		venous	18.8/10,000	
Raffini et al. [24]	2009	7 years (2001–2007)	USA national data-base (pediatric health information system)	birth to 18 years	venous	2001: 34/10,000 2007: 58/10,000	
Sandoval et al. [25]	2008	14-year period (1992–2001: group I) (2002–2005: group II)	single-centre retro-spective analysis	birth to 17 years	venous	1992: 0.3/10,000 2005: 28.8/10,000	
Tuckuviene et al. [26]	2011	12 years (1994–2006)	Denmark populati-on based study	birth to 18 years	venous and arterial non-cerebral		venous 20.9/10,000 children arterial 2.9/10,000 children

thrombosis also implicates increased disturbance of the blood vessel wall. Left-sided catheters need to be guided around more corners during insertion and hence likely do more endothelial damage (fig. 1) [1]. Male et al. [1] reported the rate of thrombosis for left- versus right-sided jugular CVADs in children is almost doubled. The relationship of thrombosis with catheter infection also suggests inflammatory changes in the blood constituents or local blood vessel wall are important. However, the relationship of the size of the catheter to the rate of thrombosis and the increased frequency of CVAD related thrombosis in smaller children, suggests that direct impedance of laminar blood flow is an important component of the pathophysiology of CVAD related thrombosis.

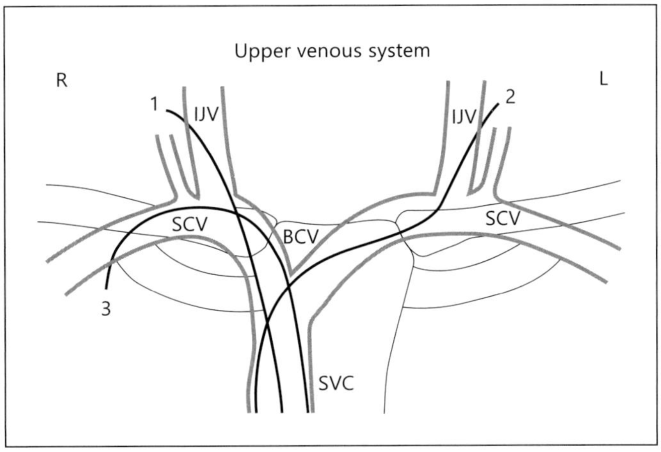

Fig. 1. The difference in pathways of insertion for left- vs. right-sided jugular CVADs. Catheters placed on the left side must traverse more corners and hence increase the risk of vascular endothelial damage, potentially explaining the notable increased rate of thrombosis for catheters placed on the left side. Reproduced with permission from Male et al. [1].

Table 2. Abnormalities in local blood flow known to be involved in the causation of venous thrombosis in neonates and children

Site	Genetic/congenital	Environmental
Upper venous system (internal jugular, axillary, subclavian, brachiocephalic veins and superior vena cava)	subclavian webs thoracic outlet syndrome (additional rib, fibrous bands, muscular development)	central vascular access devices (CVADS) percutaneous indwelling central catheters (PICCS) intravenous pacemaker wires intrathoracic tumours cardiac surgery Lemierre's syndrome (infective thrombophlebitis of the jugular vein with fusobacterium; can occur in teenagers as a post-tonsillitis phenomenon)
Intracardiac	valvular disease congenital heart disease congenital cardiomyopathy	cardiac surgery especially shunts central vascular access devices endocardial pacemaker wires cardiomyopathy atrial arrhythmias
Lower venous systems (popliteal, femoral, iliac veins, and inferior vena cava)	absent infra-renal inferior vena cava duplex inferior vena cava	central venous access devices (including umbilical vein catheters, cardiac angiography) abdominal or pelvic tumours pregnancy
Specific organ venous drainage		post-organ transplant venous stenosis (liver or kidney commonly) portal lymphadenopathy
Cerebral venous sinuses	arterio-venous malformations	mastoiditis interventional procedures (e.g. coiling) for arteriovenous malformations

An important consideration with respect to abnormalities of blood flow and thrombosis in neonates and children is that in many instances an abnormality in blood flow may not contribute to the cause of the thrombosis, but has a massive influence on the outcome of the thrombosis. The presence of right to left intracardiac shunts, and hence the possibility of paradoxical embolus, is much more common in neonates (patent foramen ovale) and in children with congenital heart disease, which constitute a large group of children at risk from thrombosis for multiple iatrogenic reasons, compared to adults. For example, a central venous line-associated thrombosis, in a child who has undergone a Norwood procedure (and thus will have a common outflow tract from their single cardiac ventricle, with pulmonary blood flow diverted via a Blalock Taussig shunt) has direct access to the systemic circulation and so the risk of paradoxical embolus and stroke is significant. Another important example is seen in children who have undergone a Fontan procedure, the definitive palliative surgery for children with univentricular cardiac physiology. The pulmonary blood flow is driven entirely by the pressure of systemic venous return, as the inferior vena cava and superior vena cava are connected directly to the pulmonary arteries. This blood flow does not increase the risk of pulmonary embolus secondary to a central line associated thrombus. However, it makes the child less tolerant to any increases in pulmonary vascular resistance, as there is no mechanism to overcome any increase in pulmonary vascular resistance (without a right ventricle in sequence), such that smaller pulmonary emboli will have a much more devastating effect in terms of capacity to maintain oxygenation through adequate pulmonary blood flow.

Abnormalities of the Blood Vessel Wall

The blood vessel wall is the component of Virchow's triad which we arguably know the least about due to the difficulties in assessing its in vivo functioning. Like the blood constituents, it would appear that the vessel wall changes with age, and there is evidence to support that the vessel wall is different in each individual vascular bed, making generalisations about the functioning of this organ system very difficult. In terms of thrombotic potential there are few clinically relevant genetic abnormalities of the blood vessel wall, with the exception of the rare connective tissue disorders such as Marfan syndrome and Ehlers Danlos syndrome. The overall clinical phenotype of these diseases usually presents before any thrombotic complications. However, many environmental precipitants may impact on the pathogenesis of thrombosis via actions on the local blood vessel wall, including CVADs as previously described. Systemic disturbances of the blood vessel wall function such as disseminated intravascular coagulation (DIC) are perhaps the more important disorders to consider under this heading. While the impact of DIC is often measured through tests of the blood constituents (APTT, INR, fibrinogen, D-dimers), it must be remembered that DIC is primarily a disease of the vascular endothelium. In numerical terms, the most common abnormality of the blood vessel wall contributing to thrombosis in children is in fact

Table 3. Incidence of venous thrombosis reported in different types of childhood cancers

Type of cancer	Patients with thromboembolism/total number of patients			
	Studies			
	Wermes et al. [27]	Knofler et al. [28]	Glaser et al. [29]	total (%)
Acute lymphoblastic leukaemia	6/73	4/25	1/3	11/101 (10.8)
Acute myeloid leukaemia	0/11	1/5	–	1/16 (6.2)
Lymphoma	2/12	3/19	3/7	8/38 (21.0)
Sarcoma	1/14	2/15	2/4	5/32 (15.6)
Neuroblastoma	0/11	0/3	1/2	1/16 (6.2)
Wilms' tumour	0/4	0/4	3/3	3/7 (42.8)
Brain tumour	1/10	–	0/1	1/11 (9.09)
Other solid tumours	–	1/6	–	1/6 (16.6)

the presence of an artificial circulatory circuit. Cardiopulmonary bypass is a crucial tool to enable modern-day management of congenital heart disease and is commonly associated with both bleeding and clotting complications. The use of ECMO (extracorporeal membrane oxygenation) and VADs (ventricular assist devices) as bridges to more definitive therapies in critically unwell children is increasing in frequency, as is the duration for which children are being maintained on these complex modalities. Haemodialysis is also a frequent therapy in tertiary paediatric care that is associated with thrombotic complications. The management of these complex modalities now takes an ever-increasing effort from haematologists, in conjunction with cardiac and intensivist teams within tertiary paediatric centres [2].

Finally, cancer is multifactorial in its contribution to the pathogenesis of thrombosis. The frequency of thrombosis varies with the type of cancer (table 3), and the treatment modalities, especially different chemotherapy regimens. Studies in children show that even for acute lymphoblastic leukaemia, the type of steroid given, and its timing in terms of concurrent asparaginase therapy, dramatically changes the thrombosis rate. Cancers likely impact on vascular endothelial function, both locally and systemically. In addition, steroids are known to impact on many factors, including vascular endothelium released or mediated molecules [3, 4].

Abnormalities of the Blood Constituents

Abnormalities of the blood constituents are the most commonly thought of aspects of Virchow's triad. In particular, there has been intense interest over the years in the respective roles of the genetic deficiencies of antithrombin (AT), protein C (PC) and protein S (PS), and more recently the factor V Leiden (FVL) and prothrombin gene mutations. Genetic abnormalities in numerous other plasma proteins have been proposed as thrombophilic risk factors, including homocysteine. However, most of these

Table 4. Proposed classification system for inherited thrombophilic conditions, routine testing methodologies, and reported frequencies in normal populations [30]

Disorders		Tests available	Population frequencies, %
Group 1 disorders (loss of function)	antithrombin deficiency	functional or antigenic assay	0.2
	protein C deficiency	functional or antigenic assay	0.2
	protein S deficiency	functional or antigenic assay	0.03–0.13
Group 2 disorders (gain of function)	activated protein C resistance	clotting assay	5
	factor V Leiden	polymerase chain reaction	5
	prothrombin gene mutation	polymerase chain reaction	2–3
	elevated levels of factors VIII, IX and XI	clotting assay	
Other disorders	hyperhomocysteinaemia	high-performance liquid chromatography	

candidates have not undergone careful segregation or population studies to define their pathogenic role. In fact, some of the seemingly obvious candidates such as abnormalities in fibrinolysis do not appear to confer thrombotic risk. These latter studies are however hampered by the low prevalence of most of these inherited abnormalities in the general population.

The most common acquired abnormality of the plasma proteins associated with thrombosis is the presence of antiphospholipid antibodies and lupus anticoagulants, although other acquired abnormalities of plasma proteins are reported. The role of antiphospholipid antibodies in children is confused by the fact that they often occur as transient phenomena, associated with infection, and in those instances are not usually associated with thrombosis. Abnormalities of the cellular components of blood are less commonly implicated, in children at least, as direct causative agents for thrombosis. Whether there are fundamental differences in the binding properties of platelets, leukocytes or other cellular components in childhood compared to adults remains to be proven.

The role of these congenital prothrombotic states (table 4) in childhood thrombosis remains controversial. The effect of more severe deficiencies has long been evident from the severely affected neonates with homozygous PC and PS deficiency [5]. How-

Fig. 2. Thrombosis-free survival in patients with hereditary thrombophilia. Note the negligible rates of thrombosis during childhood, similar to those with no thrombophilia. APCR = Activated protein C resistance. Reproduced with permission from Crowther and Kelton [30].

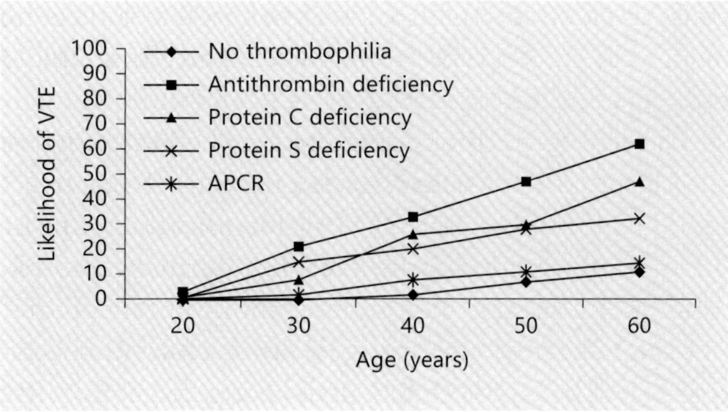

ever, the role of the heterozygous states in deep venous thrombosis during childhood is far less clear. The reported incidence of congenital prothrombotic disorders in children with venous thrombosis varies from <1% to over 60%. There have been two recent systematic reviews and meta-analyses including these and other observational studies in paediatric patients with deep venous thrombosis (DVT) and cerebrovascular occlusion (cerebral venous thrombosis and stroke), respectively [6, 7]. A third systematic review considered the role of antiphospholipid antibodies in childhood thrombosis [8].

The pooled odds ratio (OR) showed statistically significant associations between inherited thrombophilia (IT) including factor V G1691A (FVL), factor II G20210A, PC, PS, or AT deficiency, elevated lipoprotein(a), or a combination of the above factors and the presence of acquired lupus anticoagulants/antiphospholipid antibodies and venous thromboembolism (VTE) onset. The pooled odds ratios, single IT, for VTE onset ranged from 2.4 for the factor II G20210A mutation to 9.4 in children with AT deficiency. In addition, the pooled OR with respect to persistent (present on more than 2 occasions greater than 3 months apart) antiphospholipid antibodies/lupus anticoagulants was 6.6 for cerebrovascular venous occlusion and 4.9 for VTE.

However, there were many limitations with these reviews, or more specifically limitations with the quality of the observational studies that contributed data towards them. The major reasons why many experts are still dubious about the role of congenital thrombophilia in childhood thrombosis are as follows. First, if one considers the deficiencies of AT, PC, PS in addition to the FVL and prothrombin gene mutations, large family studies found negligible rates of thrombosis in children less than 15 years. This concept is illustrated in figure 2. Second, the variation in results of studies with a higher frequency of studies with better methodology finding no relationship between thrombophilia and thrombosis in most children [9, 10]. In addition, a number of cohort studies for example have failed to identify AT deficiency in children with both arterial and venous thromboembolism (TE), despite all the evidence that AT deficiency is the most severe of the inherited thrombophilias. There is similar disparity between studies concerning thrombophilia and childhood stroke. The variability in incidence reported in all these studies reflects small sample sizes, variability in study design, differing definitions of prothrombotic disorders, and different patient selection [11]. The normal variation of coagulation parameters, a phenomenon described as development haemostasis, contributes to misdiagnosis of many children, who are falsely labelled as having inherited thrombophilia. This misclassification has clearly contributed to some of the differences in published rates of inherited thrombophilia in children [12]. With the exception of teenagers with spontaneous thrombosis, few children develop thrombosis due to a heterozygous congenital prothrombotic condition, without also having an acquired risk factor. Over 80% of neonates and 70% of children with thrombosis have an acquired clinical risk factor associated with the development of the thrombosis [6–8]. Given that congenital thrombophilia is usually defined as a positive family history, combined with an early age of onset of TE, recurrent disease, and multiple or unusual locations of thrombosis, the fact that most thrombosis diagnosed in children with thrombophilia occurs in the same distribution as children with no thrombophilia and with similar clinical risk factors for thrombosis suggests that the clinical risk factors are indeed the major pathophysiological driver of thrombosis in children.

Implications for Management of Venous Thrombosis in Neonates and Children

The diagnosis of venous thrombosis in neonates and children is usually radiological and careful choice of appropriate radiological methodology is required.

Little is known about the precision and accuracy of non-invasive imaging techniques in neonates. The low pulse pressure and small vessels in premature newborns likely makes ultrasound more difficult to interpret. Similarly, the presence of CVLs makes compressibility difficult to assess, which greatly reduces the sensitivity of ultrasound. In neonates with umbilical vein catheters, Doppler ultrasound was shown to be poor compared to contrast venography in detecting asymptomatic thrombi.

The exception is renal vein thrombosis, where ultrasound is the radiographic test of choice because of its sensitivity to an enlarged kidney, as distinct from the ability to detect intravascular thrombosis. Otherwise, venography remains the gold standard where possible. Clinicians will often be forced to use a combination of clinical assessment and suboptimal imaging to make clinical decisions, because the gold standard is practically unachievable. This must be factored into progressive decision making.

In older children, there are a few more data about diagnostic strategies [13, 14]. Ultrasound was demonstrated to have a sensitivity of only 20% for intrathoracic thrombosis, yet was able to diagnose jugular thrombi that were missed on venography. There are no studies determining the sensitivity and specificity of diagnostic testing for lower venous system CVL-related thrombosis in children.

In summary, for children with suspected upper system thrombosis, a combination of ultrasound (jugular veins) and bilateral upper limb venography (subclavian and central veins) is recommended. The temptation to extend ultrasound imaging below the clavicles should be resisted. Magnetic resonance venography may be a viable alternative to formal venography depending on local expertise. For children with suspected lower system thrombosis, ultrasound is a reasonable alternative for veins distal to the groin, based on adult experience. As in adults, serial ultrasound may be required to exclude thrombosis in specific circumstances. For more proximal veins, venography or magnetic resonance venography should be considered. Of importance, while there is considerable literature about the value of sensitive D-dimer assays in excluding DVT in adults, there are no such data in children. Furthermore, given the preceding medical and surgical therapies that most children with DVT have received, D-dimer is unlikely to be of use as levels rise with trauma, surgery and cancer for example. At this time, D-dimer is not part of the recommended diagnostic strategy for venous thrombosis in children.

Careful history and examination will identify predisposing clinical risk factors and in general these should be dealt with to reduce the stimulus for further thrombosis. In particular, CVADs may need to be removed depending on the clinical circumstances. Often, when vascular access remains critical to the child's overall management, and the CVAD remains functional, then it should be left in place, despite being complicated by thrombosis. Obviously, adequate anticoagulant therapy is required whether the CVAD is removed or not. However, when considering removal of CVAD, the potential for precipitating pulmonary or paradoxical emboli is real, and often a period of anticoagulation prior to CVAD removal is recommended [15].

Screening for congenital prothrombotic disorders in children with venous TEs is of unproven benefit, regardless of the presence or absence of acquired risk factors. At this time, uniform screening of children with major illnesses, or who require CVLs, for congenital prothrombotic disorders in order to provide prophylactic therapy cannot be recommended.

Similarly, there are few data to support that the presence or absence of congenital thrombophilia should alter the principles of management. In general, anticoagulation is the mainstay of treatment for venous thromboembolism in children, with limited and very specific roles for thrombolytic therapy or surgical interventions [15]. Certainly, the intensity of treatment should not be altered by the presence of congenital thrombophilia, and duration of therapy is usually determined by the presence or absence of clinical risk factors, and the ability to modify those risk factors.

Conclusions

Environmental risk factors seem far more important to the aetiology, presentation, and management of thrombosis in children than do genetic factors. One cannot conclude that genetic factors play no role; however, the available evidence supports that in a multi-hit causation model, the major causative factors for thrombosis in children are acquired clinical, pathological and iatrogenic factors. Thus, in managing thrombosis in children, it is the amelioration of these factors that are the most important. However, there remains much to be learnt about the interaction of the coagulation system in children and the pathogenesis of thrombosis.

References

1 Male C, Chait P, Andrew M, Hanna K, Julian J, Mitchell L: Central venous line-related thrombosis in children: association with central venous line location and insertion technique. Blood 2003;101:4273–4278.

2 Chen JM, Richmond ME, Charette K, et al: A decade of pediatric mechanical circulatory support before and after cardiac transplantation. J Thorac Cardiovasc Surg 2012;143:344–351.

3 Tuckuviene R, Christensen AL, Chan AK, Athale U: Body mass index and thromboembolism in children with hematological malignancies. Pediatr Blood Cancer 2012;59:320–322.

4 Halton J, Nagel K, Brandao L, et al: Do children with central venous line (CVL) dysfunction have increased risk of symptomatic thromboembolism compared to those without CVL dysfunction, while on cancer therapy? BMC Cancer 2012;12:314.

5 Chalmers E, Cooper P, Forman K, et al: Purpura fulminans: recognition, diagnosis and management. Arch Dis Child 2011;96:1066–1071.

6 Young G, Albisetti M, Bonduel M, et al: Impact of inherited thrombophilia on venous thromboembolism in children: a systematic review and meta-analysis of observational studies. Circulation 2008;118:1373–1382.

7 Kenet G, Lutkhoff LK, Albisetti M, et al: Impact of thrombophilia on risk of arterial ischemic stroke or cerebral sinovenous thrombosis in neonates and children: a systematic review and meta-analysis of observational studies. Circulation 2010;121:1838–1847.

8 Kenet G, Aronis S, Berkun Y, et al: Impact of persistent antiphospholipid antibodies on risk of incident symptomatic thromboembolism in children: a systematic review and meta-analysis. Semin Thromb Hemost 2011;37:802–809.

9 Revel-Vilk S, Chan A, Bauman M, Massicotte P: Prothrombotic conditions in an unselected cohort of children with venous thromboembolic disease. J Thromb Haemost 2003;1:915–921.

10 van Ommen CH, Heijboer H, van den Dool EJ, Hutten BA, Peters M: Pediatric venous thromboembolic disease in one single center: congenital prothrombotic disorders and the clinical outcome. J Thromb Haemost 2003;1:2516–2522.

11 Sutor AH: Screening children with thrombosis for thrombophilic proteins. Cui bono? J Thromb Haemost 2003;1:886–888.

12 Ignjatovic V, Kenet G, Monagle P: Developmental hemostasis: recommendations for laboratories reporting pediatric samples. J Thromb Haemost 2012;10:298–300.

13 Male C, Chait P, Ginsberg JS, et al: Comparison of venography and ultrasound for the diagnosis of asymptomatic deep vein thrombosis in the upper body in children: results of the PARKAA study. Prophylactic antithrombin replacement in kids with ALL treated with asparaginase. Thromb Haemost 2002;87:593–598.

14 Shankar KR, Abernethy LJ, Das KS, et al: Magnetic resonance venography in assessing venous patency after multiple venous catheters. J Pediatr Surg 2002;37:175–179.

15 Monagle P, Chan AK, Goldenberg NA, et al: Antithrombotic Therapy in Neonates and Children: Antithrombotic Therapy and Prevention of Thrombosis, ed 9. American College of Chest Physicians Evidence-Based Clinical Practice Guidelines. Chest 2012;141(2 suppl):e737S–e801S.

16 Andrew M, David M, Adams M, et al: Venous thromboembolic complications (VTE) in children: first analysis of the Canadian registry of VTE. Blood 1994;83:1251–1257.

17 van Ommen CH, Heijboer H, Buller HR, Hirasing RA, Heijmans HS, Peters M: Venous thromboembolism in childhood: a prospective two-year registry in The Netherlands. J Pediatr 2001;139:676–681.

18 Gibson B, Chalmers E, Bolton-Maggs P, Henderson D, Lynne R: Thromboembolism in childhood: a prospective two-year BPSU study in the United Kingdom. Br J Haematol 2004;125(suppl1):1–72.

19 Newall F, Wallace T, Crock C, et al: Venous thromboembolic disease: a single-centre case series study. J Paediatr Child Health 2006;42:803–807.

20 Schmidt B, Andrew M: Neonatal thrombosis: report of a prospective Canadian and international registry. Pediatrics 1995;96:939–943.

21 Nowak-Gottl U, von Kries R, Gobel U: Neonatal symptomatic thromboembolism in Germany: two year survey. Arch Dis Child Fetal Neonatal Ed 1997; 76:F163–F167.
22 Wright JM, Watts RG: Venous thromboembolism in pediatric patients: epidemiologic data from a pediatric tertiary care center in Alabama. J Pediatr Hematol Oncol 2011;33:261–264.
23 Setty BA, O'Brien SH, Kerlin BA: Pediatric venous thromboembolism in the United States: a tertiary care complication of chronic diseases. Pediatr Blood Cancer 2012;59:258–264.
24 Raffini L, Huang YS, Witmer C, Feudtner C: Dramatic increase in venous thromboembolism in children's hospitals in the United States from 2001 to 2007. Pediatrics 2009;124:1001–1008.
25 Sandoval JA, Sheehan MP, Stonerock CE, Shafique S, Rescorla FJ, Dalsing MC: Incidence, risk factors, and treatment patterns for deep venous thrombosis in hospitalized children: an increasing population at risk. J Vasc Surg 2008;47:837–843.
26 Tuckuviene R, Christensen AL, Helgestad J, Johnsen SP, Kristensen SR: Pediatric venous and arterial noncerebral thromboembolism in Denmark: a nationwide population-based study. J Pediatr 2011;159: 663–669.
27 Wermes C, von Depka Prondzinski M, Lichtinghagen R, Barthels M, Welte K, Sykora KW: Clinical relevance of genetic risk factors for thrombosis in paediatric oncology patients with central venous catheters. Eur J Pediatr 1999;158(suppl 3):S143–S146.
28 Knofler R, Siegert E, Lauterbach I, et al: Clinical importance of prothrombotic risk factors in pediatric patients with malignancy – impact of central venous lines. Eur J Pediatr 1999;158(suppl 3):S147–S150.
29 Glaser DW, Medeiros D, Rollins N, Buchanan GR: Catheter-related thrombosis in children with cancer. J Pediatr 2001;138:255–259.
30 Crowther MA, Kelton JG: Congenital thrombophilic states associated with venous thrombosis: a qualitative overview and proposed classification system. Ann Intern Med 2003;138:128–134.

Prof. Paul Monagle, MD, MBBS, MSc, FCCP, FRCPA, FRACP
Department of Clinical Haematology
Department of Paediatrics, University of Melbourne, Royal Children's Hospital
Flemington Rd. Parkville, VIC 3052 (Australia)
E-Mail paul.monagle@rch.org.au

Thomas AE, Halsey C (eds): Controversies in Pediatric and Adolescent Hematology.
Pediatr Adolesc Med. Basel, Karger, 2014, vol 17, pp 42–66 (DOI: 10.1159/000350346)

Hematological Problems in Pediatric Intensive Care

Shoshana Revel-Vilk[a] · Peter Cox[b, d] · Nancy Robitaille[f] · Victor Blanchette[c, e]

[a]Pediatric Hematology Center, Pediatric Hematology/Oncology Department, Hadassah Hebrew University Hospital and Department of Pediatrics, Hebrew University, Jerusalem, Israel; [b]Department of Critical Care and [c]Pediatric Thrombosis and Hemostasis Program, Division of Hematology/Oncology, Hospital for Sick Children and Departments of [d]Anaesthesia and [e]Pediatrics, University of Toronto, Toronto, Ont., and [f]Blood Bank and Hemoglobinopathy Program, Division of Hematology/Oncology, CHU Sainte-Justine and Department of Pediatrics, Université de Montréal, Montréal, Que., Canada

Abstract

Hematologic abnormalities are common in children admitted to pediatric intensive care units (PICUs). Some are primary and related to the underlying hematologic disease in the child such as severe anemia in a young child with sickle cell disease and an acute splenic sequestration crisis. Others are secondary to other underlying conditions such as disseminated intravascular coagulation secondary to sepsis. Perhaps the most common association is with surgery or following trauma. The approach to the diagnosis and management of hematologic disorders in children cared for in PICUs requires an appreciation of disorders, some very rare, where delays in diagnosis and initiation of effective treatment can be associated with significant morbidity/mortality (e.g. thrombotic thrombocytopenic purpura, hemophagocytic lymphohistiocytosis) as well as more 'mundane' but equally important decisions such as transfusion triggers for replacement of packed red blood cells, fresh-frozen plasma, cryoprecipitate or platelets. In all situations, a best practice approach based on available published evidence and expert opinion is recommended. In large tertiary/quaternary care centers, a close working relationship between the pediatric intensivist staff and the clinical/laboratory hematology services is essential for optimizing the care of critically ill children with hematologic problems cared for in PICUs.
Copyright © 2014 S. Karger AG, Basel

A wide range of hematologic problems occur in patients admitted to pediatric intensive care units (PICUs). These may reflect primary hematologic disorders or arise as complications of other underlying conditions. The aim of this chapter is to focus on hematologic disorders seen in children aged >4 months to <18 years of age admitted to PICUs with an emphasis on conditions that are common or present challenges in diagnosis or management to the pediatric intensivist. For problems in neonates and younger infants (ages 0–4 months), the reader should consult other sources.

Disorders of Red Blood Cells

Anemia

Anemia is a condition in which the hemoglobin level, as a surrogate marker for the circulating red blood cell (RBC) mass, is below normal for age. An important caveat, particularly relevant to the ICU setting, is that in situations of clinically significant acute blood loss the correlation between the circulating hemoglobin level and the circulating RBC mass is often poor. In such situations the decision to transfuse donor RBCs should take into consideration other clinical parameters such as the cardiorespiratory status of the patient and other factors affecting tissue oxygenation.

Bone marrow failure (BMF), hemolysis and blood loss are the three main mechanisms that lead to anemia severe enough to need admission to the PICU. Children with severe acute or chronic anemia leading to congestive heart failure, disseminated intravascular coagulation (DIC), those with complications of inherited or acquired severe BMF states and children with sickle cell disease (SCD) presenting with certain crises (e.g. stroke, acute splenic sequestration and chest crises) are frequently managed in the PICU. The clinical findings and management of such patients are dependent on the rate at which the anemia develops, the capacity of the cardiopulmonary system to compensate and the underlying disorder or disorders that resulted in anemia.

Approximately one-half of children admitted to PICUs with anemia will receive RBC transfusions, most within the first 48 h, reflecting events such as blood loss associated with surgery and/or trauma preceding the admission [1]. Importantly, after the first 48 h, iatrogenic blood loss for laboratory testing is a significant contributor to the need for RBC transfusion in PICU, especially in young children <10 kg body weight.

There are well documented complications associated with RBC transfusions, including transfusion-transmitted infections, transfusion-related acute lung injury, transfusion-associated circulatory overload, acute hemolysis, allergic reactions and transfusion-induced immune modulation. Given the frequency of anemia in children admitted to PICUs and the potential adverse effects of RBC transfusions, a decision to transfuse RBCs should be based on the individual patient characteristics rather than a predetermined hemoglobin level [2, 3] (table 1a). Despite the very low risk of transmitting HIV or hepatitis C infection (the absolute risk may be different between countries), recent emphasis is appropriately directed toward minimizing the amount of RBC transfusions in PICU patients.

Table 1. Use of blood products in children admitted to PICU (see more details in the text)

a RBC transfusion

Key points

Suggested transfusion 'triggers'
- A hemoglobin transfusion threshold of 70 g/l can decrease RBC transfusion requirement without an increase in adverse outcome

Strategies to reduce RBC transfusion requirements
- Limit blood sampling for laboratory testing to that essential for the wellbeing of the child

RBC transfusion in children with SCD
- Simple or exchange RBC transfusions for arterial ischemic stroke, acute chest syndrome, multiorgan failure, splenic sequestration, perioperative, aplastic crisis
- Exchange (not simple) transfusion is recommended if the baseline hemoglobin level is >90 g/l and/or if a rapid decrease in HbS level to below 30% is required

Pediatric dose: 10–15 ml/kg of packed RBCs (10 ml/kg for units stored in CPDA-1, otherwise, 15 ml/kg for AS-1, AS-3, AS-5, SAGM units). In children >20 kg body weight the transfusion volume is rounded to the nearest number of packed RBC units.

b Granulocyte transfusion

Key points

Granulocyte transfusions are rarely used in children

Clinical efficacy of granulocyte transfusion is still uncertain/controversial

Hematology/transfusion medicine consultation is recommended if granulocyte transfusion is being considered in children with severe neutropenia who satisfy all of the following criteria:
- Very severe neutropenia (absolute neutrophil counts $<0.2 \times 10^9$/l) due to congenital or acquired bone marrow failure unresponsive to G-CSF therapy
- Proven or highly probable fungal or bacterial infection unresponsive to appropriate anti-infective therapy
- Neutrophil recovery expected within the near future and/or definitive or curative therapy (e.g. hematopoietic stem cell transplantation) is planned

Pediatric dose: 'buffy coat' preparation 10–20 ml/kg or apheresis granulocyte concentrate – 1 unit. All granulocyte preparations must be irradiated before transfusion.

c Platelet transfusion

Key points

Suggested prophylactic platelet transfusion 'triggers' for thrombocytopenia due to production failure
- In most cases a threshold of 10×10^9/l is safe and cost-effective
- Threshold of 20×10^9/l in neonates, in children with sepsis, and children with a higher bleeding risk (e.g. children with underlying bleeding disorders)
- Threshold of 30×10^9/l for children with brain tumors
- Threshold of 50×10^9/l for children requiring lumbar puncture, surgery
- Threshold of 100×10^9/l for children requiring neurosurgical procedures

Platelet refractoriness
- Defined as an inadequate rise in platelet counts as measured within 10 min to 1 h of a transfusion of an adequate number of platelets

Pediatric dose: 10–15 ml/kg or 1 U whole blood-derived platelets/per 10 kg body weight, up to the equivalent of 1 U of apheresis platelet or 5–6 U of whole blood-derived platelets.

Table 1. Continued

d Frozen plasma and cryoprecipitate transfusion

Key points For confirmed congenital factor deficiencies – Specific recombinant factor concentrate (or virally inactivated plasma derived concentrate if former not available) Indications for frozen plasma – For deficiency of factors II, V, VII, IX, X, XI when recombinant or plasma-derived, virus-inactivated factor concentrates are not available – For multiple factor deficiencies (e.g. liver failure) associated with severe bleeding – For DIC with active bleeding, prior to an invasive procedure and/or significant multiple factor deficiencies – For reversal of VKA (e.g. Warfarin) anticoagulation effect for patients who are actively bleeding or who require emergency surgery (PCC are licensed for this indication and may be used if readily available)
Pediatric dose: Frozen plasma: 15–20 ml/kg to a maximum of 3–4 U (the standard dose is 4 U of 250 ml for a 70-kg adult and 3 Units of 250 ml for a 50-kg adult)
Indications for cryoprecipitate – May be used when specific factor concentrates are unavailable for deficiency of factors VIII, von Willebrand factor, fibrinogen – Fibrinogen level of <0.5 g/l in the setting of a child who is not actively bleeding or <1.0 g/l in an actively bleeding child or one in whom an invasive procedure is planned
Pediatric dose: Cryoprecipitate: 1 U per 7–10 kg, to a maximum of 10 U.

SCD = Sickle cell disease; CPDA = citrate phosphate dextrose adenine; AS = additive solution; SAGM = saline adenine glucose mannitol; G-CSF = granulocyte-colony stimulating factor.

Strategies to minimize RBC transfusions in the PICU include reducing iatrogenic blood loss and reducing the hemoglobin threshold for RBC transfusion. There is no evidence to support prophylactic therapy with erythropoietin to prevent RBC transfusions in children admitted to PICUs. A randomized study involving 637 children admitted to PICUs with hemoglobin levels below 95 g/l revealed that a threshold of 70 g/l for RBC transfusion can decrease transfusion requirements without increased adverse outcomes [4]. A threshold of 70 g/l was also found to be safe in stabilized children with sepsis [5]. In children with acute blood loss, a rapid transfusion rate is essential to correct both the hypovolemia induced by blood loss and the loss of RBCs. A slow initial transfusion rate (3–5 ml/kg over 4 h) followed by another 5 ml/kg RBC over 4 h with close monitoring of cardiorespiratory status is generally recommended for children with severe chronic anemia in order to minimize the risk of transfusion circulatory overload. In children with warm autoimmune hemolytic anemia (AIHA), RBC transfusions should be avoided, if possible, until adequate treatment with corticosteroids (e.g. oral prednisone 2–4 mg/kg/day, maximum daily dose 180 mg) is initiated, and an adequate period of time given to assess response. Since matching of

RBC units is a problem in children with AIHA, immediate consultation with hematology and blood bank services is recommended in cases of acute AIHA where there is an urgent clinical need for RBC transfusion.

The risk of transfusion-transmitted cytomegalovirus (CMV) infection can be significantly reduced by transfusing either blood components from CMV seronegative donors or leukoreduced units. These two modalities are considered equivalent. Some jurisdictions such as Canada and the United Kingdom have implemented prestorage universal leukoreduction. It is unclear whether there is an advantage to provide CMV-seronegative components in addition to leukoreduction and local guidelines should be consulted.

Bone Marrow Failure

Bone marrow failure (BMF) in children may reflect acquired severe aplastic anemia, refractory cytopenias of childhood and inherited BMF disorders. Both inherited and acquired BMF states including aplastic anemia usually present with signs and symptoms of clinically significant thrombocytopenia (e.g. bruising and mucocutaneous bleeding such as epistaxis). Anemia and neutropenia are less frequent presenting features of BMF states in children. The diagnosis of BMF is based on bone marrow aspiration and biopsy. Physical examination may provide clues for the etiology of an inherited BMF syndrome such as typical facies and café-au-lait skin lesions in children with Fanconi anemia; however, genetic testing to exclude inherited BMF disorders should be performed even if no dysmorphic features are present. Acquired causes for BMF include both viral infections such as hepatitis, HIV and exposure to certain medications or chemical substances including benzene, inorganic arsenic, ionizing radiation and insecticides. However, in children, most cases of severe BMF are idiopathic. The initial management of children with BMF is supportive care including RBC and platelet transfusions and prevention and treatment of infections (table 1a–d) followed by hematopoietic stem cell transplant (HSCT) and/or immunosuppressive therapy.

Sickle Cell Disease

Children with SCD may require admission to a PICU due to severe life-threatening complications such as an arterial ischemic stroke (AIS), acute chest syndrome, severe anemia related to an aplastic crisis or splenic sequestration, infection and multiorgan failure. Severe infections (e.g. septicemia, meningitis, pneumonia) and multiorgan failure from encapsulated bacteria may develop due to functional hyposplenism. Children with SCD who have fever and/or other signs of infection should be given intravenous broad-spectrum antibiotics until blood culture results are available [6]. Vaso-occlusive pain crises may result in severe intractable pain requiring significant analgesic support. PICU management may be required in such cases to deal with respiratory suppression from opiate dosing.

Simple or exchange RBC transfusions are indicated for children presenting with AIS, acute chest syndrome, multiorgan failure, splenic sequestration, aplastic crisis or perioperatively [7]. Exchange (not simple) RBC transfusions are indicated in situations where a rapid decrease in HbS level to below 30% is required, or when the baseline hemoglobin exceeds 90 g/l in order to avoid increased blood viscosity. Hyperhemolysis syndrome is a rare complication of blood transfusion in patients with SCD. The onset is usually within 7 days of transfusion and is characterized by severe intravascular hemolysis, hemoglobinuria, and anemia to levels of hemoglobin lower than pretransfusion levels. Hyperhemolysis can be acute or delayed. Awareness of hyperhemolysis is important, as further transfusion may exacerbate ongoing hemolysis, worsen the degree of anemia and lead to a protracted course or even death. If present in a mild form, additional transfusion should be avoided, oral prednisone (1–2 mg/kg/day) should be started and the hemoglobin level monitored closely. If presenting with rapid severe hemolysis, the patient may require transfusion with intravenous immunoglobulin (IVIG) and corticosteroid treatment [8].

The basic principle of treatment of AIS in patients with SCD is to improve oxygen delivery to the brain. Neuroprotective measures for AIS include prevention of fever, treatment of seizures plus maintenance of normoglycemia and blood pressure. Other supportive measures include supplemental oxygen and prompt RBC transfusion. Exchange RBC transfusion is generally the preferred option. Because of the time involved to arrange an exchange transfusion, and the associated risks of fluctuating blood pressure with exchange transfusion, if the initial hemoglobin is less than 90 g/l, a simple RBC transfusion may be considered while arranging an exchange transfusion.

Acute chest syndrome (ACS) is the most frequent cause of admission to PICUs in patients with SCD, and challenges infection as the leading cause of SCD-related mortality in children with SCD [9]. Acute chest syndrome is defined as a new pulmonary infiltrate on a chest radiograph in a patient with SCD with new symptoms or signs such as fever, cough, sputum production, dyspnea or hypoxia; however, ACS is often a clinical diagnosis. A patient with fever or tachypnea (age 5 < 12 years: 30 breaths/min and 12 < 18 years: 25 breaths/min) or decreased O_2 saturation and an abnormal chest examination such as rales, decreased breath sounds or signs of consolidation should be treated for ACS [9]. Radiographic changes may lag behind clinical findings and therapy should start once a clinical diagnosis is made. If the chest examination is normal, a chest radiograph should be ordered. A new pulmonary infiltrate will confirm the diagnosis of ACS [9]. Nearly 50% of ACS occur in patients hospitalized for other causes (notably pain), and it is therefore critical that all hospitalized SCD patients be examined frequently and carefully, with specific attention to respiratory rate and effort and signs of consolidation on physical examination. If such findings are present, the patient should be continuously monitored by pulse oximetry [9]. It should be noted that supplemental oxygen may mask significant oxygen desaturation and therefore oxygen saturations in room air should be regularly recorded. Recognized etiologies for the ACS include infection, most commonly with atypical bacteria (e.g. *Chlamydia pneumoniae* and *Mycoplasma pneumoniae*) and pulmonary fat embolism arising from the bone marrow which is typically infarcted during acute pain crises in children with SCD and lung infarction [9]. Initial management should include intravenous administration of broad-spectrum antibiotics (including a macrolide antibiotic), supplemental oxygen, modest hydration and consideration of simple RBC transfusion [9]. The role of short-term corticosteroid therapy such as oral prednisone 2 mg/kg/day (maximum dose 60 mg/day) or its methylprednisolone equivalent remains controversial. Children with a history of asthma and those with wheezing on examination should receive bronchodilator therapy at least every 4 h. Patients with worsening respiratory distress and oxygen saturation should be managed in the PICU for exchange RBC transfusion and adequate cardiorespiratory support. Indications for mechanical respiratory support are similar to those for any patient in the PICU – inadequate oxygenation and inability to clear CO_2. The goals of ventilation are to achieve adequate O_2 delivery while at the same time using ventilatory settings that minimize the risk of ventilator-induced lung injury.

Acute splenic sequestration is caused by intrasplenic trapping of RBCs cells which causes a precipitous fall in hemoglobin level and the potential for hypoxic shock. Acute splenic sequestration may be defined by a decrease of at least 2 g/dl from the baseline hemoglobin concentration, evidence of increased erythropoiesis such as a markedly elevated reticulocyte count, and an acutely enlarging spleen. The immediate treatment of acute splenic sequestration is directed toward correction of an effective circulating red blood cell mass with RBCs delivered as a simple transfusion [6]. Usual practice is to transfuse a small volume of packed RBCs (i.e. 5 ml/kg) slowly with cardiorespiratory monitoring and monitoring of the hemoglobin level. Once RBC transfusion is employed, red cells sequestered in the spleen are remobilized, splenomegaly regresses, and the hemoglobin level increases often to a level greater than predicted on the basis of the volume of red blood cells administered. In cases with extreme anemia (hemoglobin level <30 g/l) and cardiorespiratory instability consideration should be given to performing a slow partial, isovolemic RBC exchange transfusion with careful monitoring of the patient in a PICU.

Disorders of White Blood Cells

Hyperleukocytosis

An elevated white blood cell (WBC) count is a common phenomenon in children in PICUs. Hyperleukocytosis, defined as a WBC $>100 \times 10^9$/l, is less frequent and may occur due to leukemia, severe infection, inflammation, *Bordetella pertussis*, and the hypereosinophilic syndrome (see below). Children with hyperleukocytosis may need admission to a PICU for complications associated with hyperviscosity such as hypoxemia, pulmonary hypertension and neurological symptoms (e.g. AIS).

Management of Hyperleukocytosis
Children with newly diagnosed acute leukemia and hyperleukocytosis are at increased risk of early mortality due to severe cerebral, pulmonary and metabolic complications. The frequency of hyperleukocytosis-related complications is higher in acute myelogenous leukemia (AML) than in acute lymphoblastic leukemia (ALL). Prompt reduction of the WBC count in these patients can be achieved by early initiation of chemotherapy or leukapheresis. As it may result in a significant increase in viscosity, transfusion should be avoided until the white cell count is reduced to $<100 \times 10^9/l$.

Currently, there are no clear guidelines on the best management of such patients and particularly when to perform leukapheresis. Empiric guidelines for the management of children with acute leukemia presenting with hyperleukocytosis have been developed at the Hospital for Sick Children, Toronto, Ont., Canada [10]; leukapheresis is recommended in all children with ALL or AML and clinical signs or symptoms of hyperleukocytosis, in asymptomatic children with ALL and a WBC $>400 \times 10^9/l$ or asymptomatic children with AML and a WBC $>200 \times 10^9/l$. In the recent guidelines from the American Society of Aphersis, leukapheresis is suggested for WBC $>400 \times 10^9/l$ in ALL patients and WBC $>100 \times 10^9/l$ in AML patients [11]. Leukapheresis is contraindicated in cases of acute promyelocytic leukemia and in children with massive intracranial hemorrhage [10]. Children requiring leukapheresis are frequently admitted to a PICU for central venous catheter (CVC) placement and close monitoring for possible metabolic, hemodynamic, cardiorespiratory and thrombotic complications [10–11].

Hyperleukocytosis is an independent predictor of death in infants with pertussis. Exchange transfusion to reduce the WBC count in infants <1 year of age should be considered; an algorithm for management of such infants has been proposed [12].

Leukopenia

A low WBC count often reflects a low number of neutrophils. Severe neutropenia, defined as an absolute neutrophil count plus band count of $<0.5 \times 10^9/l$, may be the presenting sign of fulminant bacterial infection or can result from viral infection, congenital disorders, chemotherapy or autoimmune disorders. The cause or causes of neutropenia influence the risk of infection: children with chemotherapy induced neutropenia, severe congenital neutropenia and BMF are at a higher risk for severe infection compared with children with viral induced neutropenia or autoimmune (benign) neutropenia of childhood.

Infection and Neutropenia
Despite the introduction of new broad-spectrum antibiotics and antifungal therapies, infections are the main cause of death in children with severe neutropenia. An evidence-based guideline has been published for the empiric management of fever and

neutropenia in children with cancer and/or those undergoing HSCT [13]. Children with severe infection may need admission to a PICU for hemodynamic and respiratory support. A sustained increase in neutrophil count is essential for fighting infections successfully; treatment strategies in severely neutropenic children include the use of granulocyte-colony stimulating factor (G-CSF) and, in rare and selected cases, granulocyte transfusions [14] (table 1b). The usual starting dose of G-CSF is 5 μg/kg administered subcutaneously daily with the aim of achieving absolute neutrophil plus band counts equal to or greater than 1×10^9/l, and with dose escalation based on response; in general doses of G-CSF greater than 60 μg/kg/day are not recommended and there are few data on the safety of doses above 24 μg/kg/day.

Disorders of Hemostasis

Bleeding Disorders

Major bleeding may be the cause for admission of children to PICUs (e.g. following trauma or surgery), or may arise during hospitalization in PICUs secondary to a variety of conditions such as DIC, liver and renal dysfunction, massive transfusion syndromes, anticoagulant overdose, thrombocytopenia, graft versus host disease and platelet dysfunction [15]. In addition, children with congenital bleeding disorders such as hemophilia A or B can suffer life-threatening hemorrhage and may require management on a PICU. In a male neonate or young infant presenting with an intracranial hemorrhage, hemophilia should be considered as part of the differential diagnosis.

Thrombocytopenia

Thrombocytopenia is the main risk factor for bleeding in children treated in the PICU setting [16]. The causes of thrombocytopenia reflect increased platelet destruction, decreased platelet production or a combination of both mechanisms. Management recommendations for thrombocytopenia are dependent on the underlying etiologies.

Immune thrombocytopenia (ITP) is a well-recognized hematologic disease in children that is mostly benign. Admission of children with ITP to a PICU is rarely needed and is generally associated with suspected or proven intra-organ or life-threatening bleeding (e.g. an intracranial hemorrhage). In such situations the goal should be to achieve a hemostatic platelet count as quickly as possible. A reasonable therapeutic approach is the immediate intravenous infusion of high-dose methylprednisolone (30 mg/kg, maximum dose 1 g infused over 30 min) plus a larger than usual transfusion of random donor platelets followed by an infusion of 1 g/kg of IVIG over 6–8 h [17]. IVIG and methylprednisolone can be repeated daily for up to 3 days. Failure to respond adequately to this enhanced regimen should prompt consideration of emergency splenectomy if not already performed and/or off-label use of recombinant factor VIIa (rFVIIa) [18], intravenous vincristine, or, if available, one of the new thrombopoietin-mimetic agents (e.g. romiplostim, eltrombopag) although the onset of response with these agents may take several days to a few weeks.

Drug-induced thrombocytopenia (DITP) is usually caused by accelerated platelet destruction by drug-dependent antibodies [19]. Decreased platelet production by megakaryocytes may also contribute to DITP. Three general criteria are required for suspecting the presence of DITP [19]. First, the implicated drug should bear a temporal relationship with thrombocytopenia, usually within 1 week after beginning a drug for the first time, or more quickly when exposed to the agent on an intermittent basis. Second, the platelet count nadir should be $<20 \times 10^9/l$. Third, there should not be an alternative explanation for the thrombocytopenia that is more highly probable than DITP. An updated list of drugs that may induce thrombocytopenia is available at http://www.ouhsc.edu/platelets. Most patients with DITP require no specific treatment, as their platelet counts will recover promptly following withdrawal of the offending agent, usually within 1 week or less [19]. In patients with severe thrombocytopenia (i.e. platelet count $<10 \times 10^9/l$) and/or severe bleeding, supportive use of platelet transfusions is recommended. The efficacy of other agents (e.g. IVIG, prednisone) in this setting is unclear. The management of heparin induced thrombocytopenia (HIT) is detailed below.

Non-immune destruction of platelets occurs secondary to endothelial cell damage. When the entire coagulation pathway is activated, the process is referred to as DIC. Viral infections, bacteremia/septicemia, malignancies, high-dose chemotherapy and vasculitis can result in endothelial cell damage that increases the rate of platelet clearance without full activation of the coagulation system. Vascular tumors can lead to platelet consumption and thrombocytopenia (Kasabach-Merritt syndrome).

The most effective therapeutic modality for DIC is removal, amelioration or management of the underlying disorder. However, in children with severe thrombocytopenia with ongoing bleeding, platelet transfusion support is appropriate in children with DIC. Platelet transfusions are not indicated in children with the Kasabach-Merritt syndrome, except in the setting of active bleeding or as preparation for invasive procedures, as it is felt that transfused platelets may fuel formation of microthrombi in areas of endothelial damage.

Children with severe thrombocytopenia secondary to production failure should be supported with platelet transfusions to avoid bleeding complications (table 1c). Transfused platelets are either single-unit, whole blood-derived platelets, buffy coat pools (prepared from 4 to 6 whole blood donations) or apheresis platelets. As for RBC transfusions, the complications and cost associated with platelet transfusions led to extensive research aiming to decrease platelet transfusions. In most cases, a threshold of $10 \times 10^9/l$ for prophylactic platelet transfusion is safe and cost effective [20]. A higher threshold of $20 \times 10^9/l$ to $30 \times 10^9/l$ is recommended in children with risk factors for bleeding (table 1c). Therapeutic platelet transfusions to control or prevent bleeding in the setting of trauma or surgery require higher transfusion thresholds. A threshold of $100 \times 10^9/l$ for neurosurgical procedures and between $50 \times 10^9/l$ and $100 \times 10^9/l$ for other invasive procedures or trauma is suggested [21]. Refractoriness to platelet transfusion may occur in ill children secondary to infections, DIC and splenomegaly. Occasionally, ill children needing repeated platelet transfusions may develop platelet refractoriness due to the development of HLA or platelet-specific alloantibodies. When ABO-mismatched platelets are used hemolysis due to high titer hemolysins is more of a risk. ABO-identical platelets or HLA best-matched, single-donor apheresis platelet concentrates may be used for support of alloimmunized patients with variable success (see http://www.transfusionontario.org/index.php#all, for details). For patients with platelet refractoriness and ongoing major life-threatening bleeding, several approaches may provide some benefit including: (1) infusion of small dose, frequent platelet transfusions at 4- to 8-hourly intervals. These transfusions may help to maintain vascular integrity even though there is no increase in the patient's posttransfusion platelet count; (2) IVIG 1 g/kg on 2 consecutive days with the aim of inducing blockade of the reticuloendothelial system and transiently increasing posttransfusion platelet increments, and (3) antifibrinolytic therapy (i.e. tranexamic acid, epsilon amino caproic acid) leading to clot stabilization [20]. Antifibrinolytic therapy is contraindicated in children with gross hematuria because of the risk of inducing obstructive clots in the genitourinary system. Recombinant FVIIa has been used to promote thrombin generation for life-threatening bleeding in subjects refractory to other conventional therapy [18]; however, its use is off label and there are emerging concerns about the risk of significant thrombosis.

Platelet Dysfunction

Platelet dysfunction is a common finding in children in PICUs. In most cases, acquired platelet dysfunction is attributable to toxins, medications such as aspirin and nitric oxide, exposure to extracorporeal circuits and renal dysfunction. Rarely, a child with a severe inherited platelet dysfunction such as Glanzmann thrombasthenia is admitted to the PICU for management of a major bleeding event [22]. Clinically, patients with platelet dysfunction demonstrate abnormal mucosal or cutaneous bleeding. If platelet dysfunction is suspected, platelet function studies (e.g. closure times with the platelet function analyzer (PFA-100®) or light transmission aggregometry) should be considered. The circulating platelet count, in most cases, is within the normal range. Treatment of bleeding episodes in children with platelet dysfunction includes elimination, if possible, of the cause for acquired platelet dysfunction, administration of antifibrinolytic agents such as tranexamic acid and epsilon aminocaproic acid (except in the presence of gross hematuria or DIC) [23] and, in selected cases, administration of platelets. The use of desmopressin (1-deamino-8-D-arginine vasopressin, DDAVP) for bleeding related to platelet dysfunction has also been suggested [24]. DDAVP is usually administered intravenously at a dose of 0.3 μg/kg (maximum dose 20 μg) in 50–100 ml of saline, infused over 30 min. Other routes of administration include subcutaneous injection and intranasal inhalation. DDAVP is generally well tolerated although treatment has been reported to cause facial flushing, headache and minor blood pressure reduction. Due to its antidiuretic properties DDAVP can cause severe hyponatremia and even seizures. This is particularly of concern when DDAVP is used in very young children or in very ill patients receiving replacement fluids intravenously.

Recombinant FVIIa is licensed for use in Glanzmann thrombasthenia and has been suggested for major bleeding associated with other congenital or acquired platelet disorders when other more conventional treatments have failed [25]. Although sometimes useful, this therapy has a somewhat unpredictable efficacy and requires high dosage (around 100 μg/kg) and frequent injections (every 2–3 h). Concomitant use of an antifibrinolytic agent can be useful.

Coagulation Disorders

Bleeding secondary to coagulation disorders, in particular acquired coagulopathies, is also common in the PICU. Children with pathologic bleeding should have laboratory testing to identify the abnormality or abnormalities that underlie the coagulation disorder. Basic laboratory screening tests include a complete blood count with a platelet count and examination of platelet morphology on a well-stained peripheral blood smear, a prothrombin time/international normalized ratio (PT/INR), an activated partial thromboplastin time (aPTT), a fibrinogen level, a thrombin time and renal and liver function tests. Additional tests may be needed based on the specific clinical scenario and on the results of the initial laboratory screening tests. Care should be taken to avoid sampling errors. Abnormal results can occur if the citrate tube is not completely filled, if the blood has a very high hematocrit, or by heparin contamination. To avoid heparin contamination, it is suggested to draw an adequate volume of blood from the CVC prior to sampling (the discard sample, at least 5 ml in infants and 10 ml in larger children), although this will not guarantee a contamination-free sample, or to draw a sample from a peripheral vein. In cases of coagulopathy, a heparin-free arterial catheter is useful and can help in acquiring reliable test results. For patients not receiving therapeutic heparin, testing could be repeated after in vitro heparin neutralization.

The results of the basic laboratory screening tests can help to define an underlying diagnosis and to guide treatment of bleeding secondary to an underlying coagulopathy (fig. 1). A prolonged aPTT may indicate heparin contamination or an inherited coagulopathy. A mixing test with normal plasma should be performed to exclude presence of a lupus anticoagulant, a common incidental finding in ill children, and heparin contamination. In both scenarios, there will be no significant correction of the clotting time. By contrast, correction of a prolonged aPTT in a mixing study suggests presence of an underlying factor deficiency or deficiencies. If the PT/INR is prolonged, vitamin K deficiency, liver disease or an inherited coagulopathy such as factor VII deficiency should be suspected. A prolonged PT/INR and aPTT together can be caused by a rare coagulation factor deficiency such as factor X or with afibrinogenemia but is more commonly due to an acquired disorder such as severe vitamin K deficiency, advanced liver failure and/or DIC.

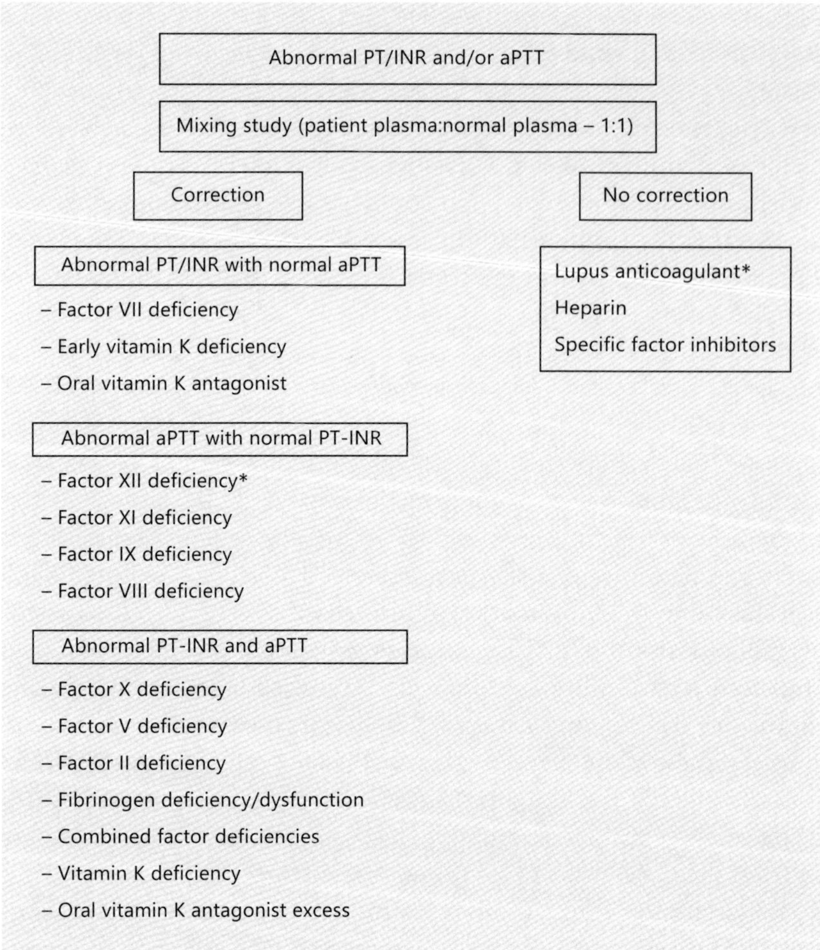

Fig. 1. Differential diagnosis of abnormal PT/INR, and aPTT. * Not associated with bleeding.

Congenital Coagulopathies

Accurate diagnosis of the underlying coagulopathy is extremely important to allow differentiation between congenital and acquired bleeding disorders so that the correct therapy can be given. Children with confirmed congenital bleeding disorders should be treated with specific recombinant or plasma-derived, virus-inactivated factor concentrates if available (table 1d). The doses and suggested target factor levels depend on the severity and site of bleeding. A hematologist expert in these disorders should be consulted. Where a specific factor replacement is not available, fresh-frozen plasma (FFP) and/or cryoprecipitate may be used (table 1d). Recombinant FVIIa has been suggested as a universal hemostatic agent [26]. This approach is not without challenges and preference should always be given to a specific replacement therapy, when available. If it is used, it is important to ensure that the patient is not acidotic or hypothermic

Table 2. Differential diagnosis of coagulopathy in patients with liver disease

Component	Vitamin K deficiency	Advanced liver failure	Disseminated intravascular coagulopathy
Coagulation factors involved	II, VII, IX, X	all factors, except factor VIII	all factors
Fibrinogen, plasma levels	normal	normal or low	low
D-dimer, plasma levels	normal	normal or elevated	elevated
Red cell morphology	normal	target cells	fragments, burrs and target cells, spherocytes
Thrombocytopenia	no	variable	yes

A practical approach for differential diagnosis includes measurement of factors V, VII and VIII plasma levels.
Low FVII with normal FV and FVIII: suggest vitamin K deficiency.
Low FVII and low FV with normal or elevated FVIII: suggest advanced liver disease.
Low FVII, low FV and low FVIII: suggest DIC.

when it is given. If rFVIIa is used it is given at a dose of ±100 μg/kg in order to optimize the likelihood of being effective. When rFVIIa is used for congenital factor VII deficiency, doses should be lower (±20 μg/kg) than the standard dose (90–270 μg/kg) used to treat bleeds in congenital FVIII or FIX complicated by the presence of inhibitors.

Acquired Coagulopathies

Liver Disease

The liver plays a central role in the hemostatic system because it produces the majority of the coagulation, anticoagulation and fibrinolytic proteins. Impaired coagulation, anticoagulation and fibrinolysis in patients with liver disease may reflect vitamin K deficiency, advanced liver failure and/or DIC (table 2). Thrombocytopenia may result from decreased production (low thrombopoietin levels), increased consumption from splenic sequestration of platelets secondary to portal hypertension and splenomegaly, and/or DIC. Platelet function defects are also reported, but are of unclear significance.

The defects in platelet number and function, procoagulant factors and regulation of fibrinolysis often are balanced by elevated FVIII and von Willebrand factor levels, deficiencies of protein C, protein S and antithrombin, natural anticoagulants, and by decreased levels of the natural inhibitors of fibrinolysis. However, this hemostatic balance is not stable and may alternate quickly between hypo- or hypercoagulable states, depending on the patient status [27]. Patients with liver disease frequently have abnormal PT/INR and aPTT tests, yet due to deficiencies in the anticoagulation factors the bleeding risk is not necessarily high. Indeed, an increased risk of thromboembolic events (TEs) has been described in patients with liver failure [28]. No screening tests can predict with confidence the bleeding risks in patients with liver failure. The role of global tests of hemostasis, such as thromboelastography or thrombin generation tests, in this setting merits further study.

There is a lack of pediatric studies to guide decision making in children with liver disease, so the majority of recommendations are based on adult guidelines [28]. Replacement of vitamin K should be considered in all patients with liver failure. In children with asymptomatic abnormal PT/INR with or without mild bleeding, the recommended dose of vitamin K is 30 μg/kg given intravenously, subcutaneously or orally [28]. Higher doses of 5 mg (0.1–0.2 mg/kg) given intravenously are suggested for children with major and life-threatening bleeding. The patient's PT/INR should be measured 2–6 h following the initial dose of vitamin K to assess response. If there is no response to an adequate trial of vitamin K (dosing daily for up to 3 days), repeated administration of large doses of vitamin K should be avoided as this may result in further depression of liver function in patients with severe liver disease. Oral vitamin K supplementation (2.5–5 mg, 2–5 times a week) is suggested for children with chronic liver disease. For children with liver failure who bleed, platelets, FFP and cryoprecipitate infusions should be considered based on the deficiencies of the different hemostatic proteins (table 1d). Use of antifibrinolytic agents should be considered in cases with laboratory evidence of a hyperfibrinolytic state. Use of prothrombin complex concentrates (PCCs) can be considered if there is failure to control bleeding with standard therapy or when patients have volume overload problems but should be used with caution because of the risk of thromboembolism. Use of off-label rFVIIa could be considered if bleeding is not controlled with adequate dose of PCCs [28].

According to the American Association for the Study of Liver Disease guidelines, platelet transfusion should be considered prior to liver biopsy when platelet counts are $<50–60 \times 10^9$/l [29]. Although many centers avoid standard percutaneous liver biopsy if the PT/INR is >1.5, strict cutoffs for PT/INR are considered inappropriate in light of the risks associated with FFP infusion and the lack of data to support a correlation between elevated PT/INRs and increased risk of bleeding in patients with liver failure [29]. Whether a new measure of coagulation in liver disease such as the 'INR_{LIVER}', which recalculates the International Sensitivity Index from a reference point of patients with liver disease rather than coumadin-treated patients [30], will provide a reliable measure of bleeding risk remains to be determined.

Disseminated Intravascular Coagulation

DIC has been defined as an acquired syndrome characterized by the intravascular activation of coagulation with loss of localization arising from different causes. It can originate from and cause damage to the microvasculature, which if sufficiently severe, can produce organ dysfunction. Conditions that may result in DIC include sepsis, trauma, malignancy and severe hepatic failure, which induce a systemic inflammatory response with activation of the cytokine network and subsequent activation of the coagulation cascade leading to release or exposure of procoagulant material into the circulation. The clinical spectrum of DIC can range from a subclinical decrease in platelet count or prolongation of the PT/INR/aPTT to fulminant DIC with widespread microvascular thrombosis and profuse bleeding. The laboratory screen in DIC may show any combination of abnormal tests: thrombocytopenia, a decreased fibrinogen level, a prolonged PT/INR, a prolonged aPTT, and elevated markers of fibrinolysis (D-dimer). These last markers are not specific for DIC and can occur in other situations such as postsurgery or in renal impairment. The diagnosis of DIC cannot be established on the basis of a single laboratory test, but requires assessment of the entire test panel. Scoring systems established to diagnose DIC in adults [31] are not yet validated in children.

The treatment of DIC involves aggressive treatment of the underlying condition and supportive care. Platelet, cryoprecipitate and FFP transfusions should only be used in children with active bleeding, those undergoing an invasive procedure or those with significant depletion of these hemostatic factors (e.g. platelets, fibrinogen, multiple factor deficiencies) (table 1d). Vitamin K deficiency can be treated with vitamin K supplementation. The role for anticoagulation and/or treatment with activated protein C in children with DIC is not proven [32] and in fact activated protein C has been withdrawn from the market due to safety concerns.

Anticoagulant Overdose

Children receiving anticoagulation may develop bleeding complications [33]. If unfractionated heparin needs to be discontinued for clinical reasons, termination of the infusion usually will suffice because of the rapid clearance of unfractionated heparin. If immediate reversal is required, protamine sulfate is used with a dose based on the amount of unfractionated heparin received in the previous 2 h [33]. The reversal of low-molecular-weight heparin (LMWH) is more problematic. There are some data to support the use of protamine sulfate. Protocols for reversal of LMWH have been published [33]. In children treated with a vitamin K antagonist (VKA) such as coumadin or warfarin, the presence of an excessively prolonged INR (usually >8.0) in a patient with no significant bleeding can be treated with vitamin K (30 μg/kg). In the presence of clinically significant bleeding, immediate reversal using PCCs or support with FFP may be required (table 1d) [33].

Thrombotic Disorders

Thromboembolic events (TEs) are a rare complication in pediatric medicine. There has, however, been an increase in the frequency of TEs in childhood over the past two decades, likely due to a true increase in incidence, an increase in detection of previously undiagnosed TEs and advances in medical expertise and technology leading to an increase in survival of children with previously fatal conditions and an increase in complications of complex conditions managed in tertiary care centers. In contrast to

Table 3. Clinical criteria for risk for VTE and bleeding in critically ill children after trauma

Risk factors for VTE	Risk factors for bleeding
Projected immobility >5 days	Intracranial bleed
Glasgow Coma Scale <9	Solid organ injury
Presence of central venous catheter	Planned surgical intervention or invasive procedure in the next 24 h
Spinal cord injury	Thrombocytopenia
Complex lower extremity fracture	Coagulopathy
Operative pelvic fracture	Renal failure
Use of inotropes	Personal and/or family history of bleeding disorder
Cardiopulmonary resuscitation	
Exogenous estrogen	
Chronic inflammatory state	
History of previous clot*	
Known thrombophilia	
Current malignancy	

High risk of VTE: age ≥13 years OR age <13 years with ≥4 risk factors for VTE.
Low risk of VTE: age <13 years AND ≤3 risk factors for VTE.
Low risk of bleeding: no risk factors for bleeding.
High risk of bleeding: one or more risk factors for bleeding.
Modified from Hanson et al. [35].
* Patients with recurrent thrombosis should be considered high risk for VTE regardless of age and/or presence of other risk factors.

adults, most TEs in children are associated with predisposing risk factors including CVCs, cardiovascular disease, surgery, infection and malignancy. The presence of a CVC or an arterial catheter is the single most important risk factor for venous and arterial TEs in children. The approach to diagnosis, including the role of laboratory thrombophilia, in children with TEs has recently been reviewed [34].

The management of TEs in children is based on limited data. Thus, where possible, it is recommended that pediatric hematologists with experience in the field of thrombosis and hemostasis should manage children with TEs. When this is not possible, a combination of a pediatrician and adult hematologist supported by consultation with an experienced pediatric hematologist is suggested [33]. The chapter on antithrombotic therapy in neonates and children of the American College of Chest Physicians Evidence-Based Clinical Practice Guidelines is updated every 4 years and is a useful resource for the management of children with TEs [33].

Routine thromboprophylaxis is currently not recommended for children with short-term CVCs, such as those used in the PICU setting [33]. Thromboprophylaxis for critically ill children following trauma should be individualized and based on the risk for venous TE (VTE) versus the risk of bleeding (table 3). Although not evidence based, a management approach was suggested based on these risks [35]. For patients at high risk of VTE with a low risk of bleeding, anticoagulation with LMWH using a dose of 0.5 mg/kg administered subcutaneously twice daily until hospital discharge has been suggested [35]. For patients at high risk of VTE and high risk for bleeding, sequential compression devices and a screening ultrasound examination of both lower extremities on PICU day 7, and of upper extremities if a CVC is present has been suggested [35]. No anticoagulation or other clinical intervention was suggested for patients at low risk of VTE. In a prospective cohort of children following trauma, implementation of these recommendations decreased the incidence of VTE without increasing the incidence of bleeding complications [35].

Catastrophic antiphospholipid syndrome is a potentially rare life-threatening condition presenting with rapidly developing multiple organ involvement, laboratory confirmation of the presence of antiphospholipid antibodies, usually in high titer, and histopathologic evidence of multiple small-vessel occlusions. Criteria for classification of catastrophic antiphospholipid syndrome have been published [36]. Children with catastrophic antiphospholipid syndrome may be admitted to PICUs due to pulmonary, cerebral and/or cardiac complications. Management includes treatment of precipitating factors, such as infections and certain medications (e.g. anticoagulation), effective anticoagulation and high-dose corticosteroid therapy [36]. In severe cases, IVIG, plasma exchange, cyclophosphamide and rituximab may be needed.

Although very rare in children, HIT has been reported to occur in the PICU setting. The classic picture of HIT is the onset of moderate thrombocytopenia approximately 1 week following exposure to heparin without an alternate explanation for the thrombocytopenia [37]. Unfortunately, this classic picture is often masked in ill children in the PICU in whom thrombocytopenia from multiple etiologies is common [38]. A diagnosis of HIT in the PICU therefore relies on an awareness of the condition plus confirmatory tests to document presence of heparin antibody platelet factor 4 (PF4) immune complexes. The management of children with suspected or proven HIT should always involve the advice of a hematologist because of the real risk of arterial/venous thrombosis in this situation [38]. If a diagnosis of HIT is strongly suspected or proven, discontinuation of all heparin is mandatory with consideration of an alternative anticoagulant (e.g. bivalirudin, argatroban or fondaparinux) that does not cross-react with HIT antibodies [38].

Miscellaneous Disorders

Thrombotic Microangiopathies (TTP and HUS)

The term thrombotic microangiopathy (TMA) refers to a developing spectrum of diseases, which are characterized by the presence of systemic microvascular thrombosis that leads to thrombocytopenia and microangiopathic anemia. Traditionally, TMA encompasses the disorders thrombotic thrombocytopenic purpura (TTP) and hemolytic uremic syndrome (HUS). However, TMAs may additionally occur in other disorders such as systemic lupus erythematosus, antiphospholipid antibody syndrome, allogeneic HSCT, disseminated malignancy and malignant hypertension, or may be triggered by various infectious agents such as bacteria (e.g. *Streptococcus pneumonia*) and viruses (e.g. influenza A H1N1). Drugs that may cause TTP include quinine, mitomycin C and cyclosporine.

Most cases of TTP are acquired and reflect autoantibody inhibition of ADAMTS13, a metalloprotease responsible for cleaving the ultra-high-molecular-weight forms of von Willebrand factor released from endothelial cells upon stimulation; rare cases are congenital (the Upshaw-Schulman syndrome) reflecting a mutation in the ADAMTS13 gene leading to marked deficiency of ADAMTS13 activity. The classic pentad of thrombocytopenia, microangiopathic hemolytic anemia, neurologic and renal abnormalities, and fever occurs in a minority (<10%) of TTP cases. Leading experts in the field of TMAs recommend urgent treatment of all cases that fulfill the current diagnostic criteria for TTP: microangiopathic hemolytic anemia and thrombocytopenia, with or without renal failure or neurological abnormalities, and without another cause for TMA [39]. Initial treatment, which can be lifesaving, includes plasma exchange using plasma as replacement fluid: all plasma products (FFP, 24-hour plasma and cryoprecipitate-poor plasma) appear to have equal efficacy [39]. Plasma exchange (1–1.5 blood volume) should be urgently started and continued daily until the platelet count has normalized for 2 days. Consolidation treatment with plasma exchange is recommended. For cases that fail to respond to initial plasma exchange therapy, or where there is clinical or laboratory deterioration on daily plasma exchange therapy, twice daily plasma exchange plus corticosteroid therapy [prednisone 1–2 mg/kg or methylprednisolone 30 mg/kg/day, maximum dose 1 g/day for 3 consecutive days and/or rituximab therapy (375 mg/m^2 weekly for 2–4 consecutive weeks)] should be considered.

Typical HUS, often described as Shiga-toxin producing *Escherichia coli* (STEC HUS), was described to occur predominantly in children [40]. Of interest, however, in the recent outbreak of HUS in Germany, 2011, mainly females in their 30/40 s were affected. Presenting features included abdominal pain, bloody diarrhea, microangiopathic hemolytic anemia, thrombocytopenia and renal failure. The abdominal pain and bloody diarrhea are manifestations of hemorrhagic enterocolitis caused by Shiga toxin-producing bacteria, in North America most commonly *E. coli* O157:H7. Treatment of STEC HUS should include supportive measures and peritoneal or hemodialysis, when needed [40]. Much less often children with HUS present without a prodrome of diarrhea, with a more aggressive course of disease and in some cases a family history of HUS. These cases are labeled as atypical HUS. The most common cause of atypical HUS are mutations in genes encoding regulation of the alternate complement pathway (loss of function mutations: CFH, CFI, MCP/CD46, THBD/CD141; and gain of function mutations: C3, CFB), or the presence of autoantibodies specifi-

Table 4. Current classification of hypereosinophilic syndrome (HES)*

Primary (clonal/neoplastic)	Myeloid and lymphoid neoplasms with eosinophilia and abnormalities of PDGFRA, PDGFRB, or FGFR1 Chronic eosinophilic leukemia, not otherwise specified WHO-defined myeloid neoplasm with associated eosinophilia Lymphocyte-variant hypereosinophilia (cytokine-producing, immunophenotypically-aberrant T cell population)
Secondary (reactive)	*Common causes:* helminth infections, allergic reactions, atopic diseases, drug reactions (allergic or toxic) *Rare causes:* chronic graft-versus-host disease, Hodgkin lymphoma, B or T cell lymphoma/leukemia, Langerhans cell histiocytosis, indolent systemic mastocytosis, solid tumors/malignancy, scabies, other infestations, allergic bronchopulmonary aspergillosis, chronic inflammatory disorders, autoimmune diseases
Idiopathic HES	No underlying cause of hypereosinophilia identified, no evidence of a reactive or neoplastic condition/disorder underlying hypereosinophilia

* HES is defined as blood hypereosinophilia with end-organ damage attributable to tissue hypereosinophilia.
PDGFRA, PDGFRB = Platelet-derived growth factor receptor alpha/beta; FGFR1 = fibroblast growth factor receptor 1. Modified from Valent et al. [42].

cally binding to CFH (the presence of CFH autoantibodies is typically found in absence of CFHR1/3, a condition named DEAP-HUS) [41]. These children often have recurrent episodes of HUS. Current opinion supports use of plasma exchange in cases of atypical HUS. A new treatment for children with atypical HUS is eculizumab, a humanized monoclonal anti-C5 antibody that inhibits complement factor 5 (C5) thus preventing the induction of the terminal complement cascade including the formation of the membrane attack complex C5b-9 [41].

Hypereosinophilia

Hypereosinophilia, defined as an absolute eosinophil count of $>1.5 \times 10^9$/l, is a disorder associated with allergic, infectious, malignant and systemic inflammatory diseases. Depending on the underlying etiology eosinophilia varies in severity from a self-limiting, benign disorder to a life-threatening illness involving critical organs such as the heart, lung and brain [42, 43]. The 2011 Working Conference on Eosinophilic Disorders and Syndromes updated the criteria and definitions for eosinophilic disorders [42]. After exclusion of secondary (reactive) causes of eosinophilia (table 4), the workup should proceed to the evaluation of a primary bone marrow disease [43]. Lymphocyte-variant hypereosinophilia is a mixture of clonal and reactive process;

clonal T cells are identified as the potential cause. Prompt identification of clonal disorders is important and has therapeutic implications. Idiopathic hypereosinophilic syndrome is a diagnosis of exclusion when no underlying cause in identified and hypereosinophilia-related organ damage is present. Certain rare syndromic disorders associated with hypereosinophilia are described (e.g. Churg-Strauss, Gleich, Omenn, hyper-IgE and eosinophilia myalgia syndromes) [42].

An algorithm for investigation and management of hypereosinophilia has been proposed [43]. Evidence of eosinophilia-associated organ dysfunction or damage (e.g. mural thrombi in the heart), or neurologic impairment requires prompt therapy with corticosteroids plus, in selected cases, other agents including hydroxyurea and interferon-α. Imatinib mesylate is considered front-line therapy in cases of hypereosinophilia with re-arrangements of the platelet-derived growth factor receptor (PDGFR) A/B or fibroblast growth factor receptor (FGFR1) genes. The use of steroids is applicable for hypereosinophilic syndrome without FIP1L-PDGFRA fusion. The role of humanized anti-IL5 monoclonal antibody (mepolizumab) and anti-CD52 (alemtuzumab) antibody therapy remains investigational.

Hemophagocytic Lymphohistiocytosis

Hemophagocytic lymphohistiocytosis (HLH) is a potentially fatal hyperinflammatory syndrome with prolonged fever, hepatosplenomegaly and the characteristic laboratory findings of anemia and thrombocytopenia, hypofibrinogenemia, hypertriglyceridemia and hyperferritinemia. Prompt initiation of therapy is essential for survival, but timely diagnosis may be challenging due to the rarity of HLH, its variable presentation, non-specific clinical findings, and the time required to perform diagnostic testing. The accepted incidence of HLH is 1 per 3,000 in-patient admissions [44]. The major pathogenetic factors underlying HLH include loss of cytotoxic T cells (CTL) and natural killer (NK) cell function which allows prolonged antigen stimulation, leading to hyperactivation of T lymphocytes and macrophages, proliferation and infiltration of these cells into various organs and hypercytokinemia [45]. HLH may be inherited (primary/familial) or may be secondary to any severe infection, malignancy or rheumatologic condition.

The most common symptoms of HLH are prolonged fever (>7 days), hepatosplenomegaly, jaundice, skin rash, anemia, bleeding, lymphadenopathy, ascites and edema. Liver dysfunction with transaminitis is common. The diagnosis should be considered in all patients presenting with idiopathic liver failure. Pulmonary infiltrates leading to respiratory failure and neurologic abnormalities, such as cranial nerve palsies, seizures and decreased level of consciousness are common and renal failure may also be seen but not usually in isolation. Hyponatremia and hypoalbuminemia may occur as well as elevation of D-dimers even when the PT/INR and aPTT are normal. HLH is a syndrome that is diagnosed based on clinical and labora-

Table 5. Currently used criteria for diagnosis of HLH

1	A molecular diagnosis consistent with HLH
or	
2	Five out of the eight criteria below are fulfilled
a	Fever ≥38.3°C
b	Splenomegaly
c	Cytopenias (affecting ≥2 or 3 lineages in the peripheral blood):
i	Hemoglobin <90 g/l (in infants <4 weeks: hemoglobin <100 g/l)
ii	Platelets $<100 \times 10^9$/l
iii	Neutrophils $<1.0 \times 10^9$/l
d	Hypertriglyceridemia and/or hypofibrinogenemia
i	Fasting triglycerides ≥3.0 mmol/l (≥265 mg/dl)
ii	Fibrinogen ≤1.5 g/l
e	Hemophagocytosis in bone marrow or spleen or lymph nodes
f	Low or absent NK cell activity (according to local laboratory reference)
g	Ferritin ≥500 μg/l (based on experts opinion ferritin >3,000 μg/l is concerning, >10,000 μg/l is highly suspicious for HLH)
h	Elevated soluble CD25 (soluble IL-2 receptor alpha) (according to local laboratory reference ranges)

Modified from Jordan et al. [44].

tory criteria [44] (table 5). Soluble CD25 is considered the most useful inflammatory marker, as it correlates with current disease activity more consistently than ferritin or other disease indices. However, ferritin is often a valuable marker because levels above 10,000 μg/l are highly sensitive and specific for the diagnosis of HLH. Hemophagocytosis is neither sensitive nor specific for HLH and is currently considered a less important diagnostic criterion [44]. Because not all patients have hemophagocytosis at disease onset, diagnosis should not be delayed looking for this single feature. In general, it is not one single feature but the severity of the overall picture that is important when considering a diagnosis of HLH in a child. Looking for such evidence of immunopathology, seen when immune hyperactivity results in organ damage, will prevent misdiagnosis.

Without therapy, survival of patients with active familial HLH is approximately 2 months. The principal goal of induction therapy is to suppress the life-threatening inflammatory process that underlies HLH. It is important to initiate therapy promptly even in the face of unresolved infections, cytopenias, or organ dysfunction. The current standard of care consists of a decrescendo course of cyclosporine, etoposide and dexamethasone, with or without intrathecal therapy. At the end of 8 weeks, patients are either weaned off therapy or transitioned to continuation therapy, which is intended only as a bridge to HSCT [44]. HLA typing should be sent at the start of induction therapy to avoid downstream delays in HSCT. It is not necessary to distinguish primary from secondary HLH for initiation of therapy but at some stage this distinction needs to be made as all primary HLH needs to have the defective gene replaced through HSCT. Genetic testing should be done in all young children and at any age if primary/familial HLH is suspected. It must be remembered that siblings who are potential stem cell donors may themselves have HLH which has not yet been manifest and must be tested prior to any donation. Reduced intensity conditioning for HSCT has reduced the high transplant associated mortality and is the current standard.

Supportive care guidelines for patients on therapy for HLH should be similar to standard practice for patients undergoing HSCT including acute care nursing, *Pneumocystis carinii* prophylaxis, consideration for fungal prophylaxis, IVIG supplementation and neutropenic precautions. Any new fever should be evaluated for HLH reactivation, as well as an opportunistic infection, and empiric broad spectrum antibiotic therapy initiated. Inflammation, consumptive coagulopathy, and intrinsic platelet defects may lead to very high risk of spontaneous bleeding. Ideally, critically ill patients with HLH should be treated at facilities familiar with care of cancer and bone marrow transplant patients.

Macrophage activation syndrome is a recognized major complication of certain rheumatologic disorders (e.g. juvenile idiopathic arthritis, systemic lupus erythematosus) and is thought of as a rheumatic disease associated with HLH [44]. The main clinical manifestations include fever, hepatosplenomegaly, hepatitis, lymphadenopathy and DIC. Cytopenias are a late finding. Hemophagocytosis in the bone marrow or other tissues is an important finding [44]. In patients with macrophage activation syndrome diagnosed in the context of associated rheumatologic diseases, treatment with increased immunosuppression (e.g. pulse high-dose methylprednisolone and/or high-dose IVIG) is often effective. In selected cases it may be necessary to add cyclosporine and/or other autoimmune disease-specific therapy, etoposide, other HLH salvage therapy or HSCT [44].

Conclusion

This chapter has focused on hematologic disorders where timely and accurate diagnosis is essential for achieving an optimal outcome. Guides for replacement of blood components in various clinical situations have been provided with the caveat that it is the responsibility of the physician caring for a child in the PICU setting to carefully weigh the risks and benefits of all therapeutic options, and, after consultation with the child if of an appropriate age, and their family, to select the optimal management for the given situation. Since significant changes in the clinical condition of children in PICUs is common, frequent reassessment of the child's condition based on repeated physical examination and available laboratory parameters is essential to allow optimal decision making. The recommendations in this chapter are provided with this caveat. For more detailed information, the reader should consult the references provided.

Acknowledgments

The authors wish to thank Drs. Sheila Weitzman (Division of Hematology/Oncology, the Hospital for Sick Children, Toronto, Canada), Christoph Licht (Division of Nephrology, the Hospital for Sick Children, Toronto, Canada), Hans Hitzler (Division of Hematology/Oncology, the Hospital for Sick Children, Toronto, Canada), Heather Hume (Pediatric Hematology/Oncology, CHU Sainte-Justine Montreal, Canada), Georges-Etenne Rivard (Pediatric Hematology/Oncology, CHU Sainte-Justine Montreal, Canada) and Jacques Braun (Pediatric Intensive Care Unit, Hadassah Hebrew University Hospital, Jerusalem, Israel) for their useful suggestions during the preparation of this manuscript.

References

1 Bateman ST, Lacroix J, Boven K, Forbes P, Barton R, Thomas NJ, et al: Anemia, blood loss, and blood transfusions in North American children in the intensive care unit. Am J Respir Crit Care Med 2008; 178:26–33.
2 Istaphanous GK, Wheeler DS, Lisco SJ, Shander A: Red blood cell transfusion in critically ill children: a narrative review. Pediatr Crit Care Med 2011;12: 174–183.
3 Parker RI: Red blood cell transfusions in children: treat the child, not the number! Pediatr Crit Care Med 2011;12:226–228.
4 Lacroix J, Hebert PC, Hutchison JS, Hume HA, Tucci M, Ducruet T, et al: Transfusion strategies for patients in pediatric intensive care units. N Engl J Med 2007;356:1609–1619.
5 Karam O, Tucci M, Ducruet T, Hume HA, Lacroix J, Gauvin F: Red blood cell transfusion thresholds in pediatric patients with sepsis. Pediatr Crit Care Med 2011;12:512–518.
6 National Institutes of Health Publication: The Mangement of Sickle Cell Disease, ed 4. Bethesda, National Institutes of Health Publication, 2002. http://www.nhlbi.nih.gov/health/prof/blood/sickle/sc_mngt.pdf.
7 Swerdlow PS: Red cell exchange in sickle cell disease. Hematology (Am Soc Hematol Educ Program) 2006; 2006:48–53.
8 Win N: Hyperhemolysis syndrome in sickle cell disease. Expert Rev Hematol 2009;2:111–115.
9 Miller ST: How I treat acute chest syndrome in children with sickle cell disease. Blood 2011;117:5297–5305.
10 http://www.sickkids.ca/clinical-practice-guidelines/clinical-practice-guidelines/Management-of-Children-with-Acute-Leukemia-and-an-Elevated-WBC-at-Diagnosis.html.
11 Szczepiorkowski ZM, Winters JL, Bandarenko N, Kim HC, Linenberger ML, Marques MB, et al: Guidelines on the use of therapeutic apheresis in clinical practice – evidence-based approach from the Apheresis Applications Committee of the American Society for Apheresis. J Clin Apher 2010;25:83–177.
12 Rowlands HE, Goldman AP, Harrington K, Karimova A, Brierley J, Cross N, et al: Impact of rapid leukodepletion on the outcome of severe clinical pertussis in young infants. Pediatrics 2010;126:e816–e827.
13 Lehrnbecher T, Phillips R, Alexander S, Alvaro F, Carlesse F, Fisher B, et al: Guideline for the management of fever and neutropenia in children with cancer and/or undergoing hematopoietic stem-cell transplantation. J Clin Oncol 2012;30:4427–4438.
14 Clinical Guidelines for the Use of Granulocyte Transfusions. 2011. http://hospital.blood.co.uk/library/pdf/inf276_2.pdf.
15 Kenet G, Strauss T, Kaplinsky C, Paret G: Hemostasis and thrombosis in critically ill children. Semin Thromb Hemost 2008;34:451–458.
16 Moorehead PC, Cyr J, Klaassen R, Barrowman NJ, Menon K: An evidence-based threshold for thrombocytopenia associated with clinically significant bleeding in pediatric intensive care unit patients. Pediatr Crit Care Med 2012;13:e316–e322.
17 Provan D, Stasi R, Newland AC, Blanchette VS, Bolton-Maggs P, Bussel JB, et al: International consensus report on the investigation and management of primary immune thrombocytopenia. Blood 2010; 115:168–186.
18 Levi M, Peters M, Buller HR: Efficacy and safety of recombinant factor VIIa for treatment of severe bleeding: a systematic review. Crit Care Med 2005; 33:883–890.
19 http://www.uptodate.com/contents/drug-induced-thrombocytopenia#H1.
20 Slichter SJ: Evidence-based platelet transfusion guidelines. Hematology (Am Soc Hematol Educ Program) 2007;2007:172–178.

21 Guideline for Platelet Transfusion Thresholds for Pediatric Hematology/Oncology Patients. 2011. http://www.c17.ca/index.php?cID=86.
22 Israels SJ, Kahr WH, Blanchette VS, Luban NL, Rivard G, Rand M: Platelet disorders in children: a diagnostic approach. Pediatr Blood Cancer 2011;56:975–983.
23 Konkle BA: Acquired disorders of platelet function. Hematology (Am Soc Hematol Educ Program) 2011; 2011:391–396.
24 Ben-Ami T, Revel-Vilk S: The use of DDAVP in children with bleeding disorders. Pediatr Blood Cancer 2013;60(suppl 1):S41–S43.
25 Poon MC: The evidence for the use of recombinant human activated factor VII in the treatment of bleeding patients with quantitative and qualitative platelet disorders. Transf Med Rev 2007;21:223–236.
26 Hoots WK: Challenges in the therapeutic use of a 'so-called' universal hemostatic agent: recombinant factor VIIa. Hematology (Am Soc Hematol Educ Program) 2006;2006:426–431.
27 Lisman T, Porte RJ: Rebalanced hemostasis in patients with liver disease: evidence and clinical consequences. Blood 2010;116:878–885.
28 Wicklund BM: Bleeding and clotting disorders in pediatric liver disease. Hematology (Am Soc Hematol Educ Program) 2011;2011:170–177.
29 Rockey DC, Caldwell SH, Goodman ZD, Nelson RC, Smith AD: Liver biopsy. Hepatology 2009;49:1017–1044.
30 Bellest L, Eschweege V, Poupon R, Chazouilleeres O, Robert A: A modified international normalized ratio as an effective way of prothrombin time standardization in hepatology. Hepatology 2007;46:528–534.
31 Taylor FB Jr, Toh CH, Hoots WK, Wada H, Levi M: Towards definition, clinical and laboratory criteria, and a scoring system for disseminated intravascular coagulation. Thromb Haemost 2001;86:1327–1330.
32 Brandao LR, Howard SC, Gow KW, Rajasekaran S, Tamurro RF: Hematology and oncology in critical illness; in Lucking SE, Maffei FA, Tamburro RF, Thomas NJ (eds): Pediatric Critical Care Study Guide. London, Springer, 2012, pp 801–850.
33 Monagle P, Chan AK, Goldenberg NA, Ichord RN, Journeycake JM, Nowak-Gottl U, et al: Antithrombotic therapy in neonates and children: antithrombotic therapy and prevention of thrombosis, ed 9. American College of Chest Physicians Evidence-Based Clinical Practice Guidelines. Chest 2012; 141(2 suppl):e737S–e801S.
34 Rizzi M, Barnes C: A diagnostic approach to a child with thrombosis; in Blanchette V, Breakey V, Revel-Vilk S (eds): SickKids Handbook of Pediatric Thrombosis and Hemosthasis. Basel, Karger, 2013.
35 Hanson SJ, Punzalan RC, Arca MJ, Simpson P, Christensen MA, Hanson SK, et al: Effectiveness of clinical guidelines for deep vein thrombosis prophylaxis in reducing the incidence of venous thromboembolism in critically ill children after trauma. J Trauma Acute Care Surg 2012;72:1292–1297.
36 Cervera R: Update on the diagnosis, treatment, and prognosis of the catastrophic antiphospholipid syndrome. Curr Rheumatol Rep 2010;12:70–76.
37 Warkentin TE: HITlights: a career perspective on heparin-induced thrombocytopenia. Am J Hematol 2012;87(suppl 1):S92–S99.
38 Takemoto CM, Streiff MB: Heparin-induced thrombocytopenia screening and management in pediatric patients. Hematology (Am Soc Hematol Educ Program) 2011;2011:162–169.
39 George JN: How I treat patients with thrombotic thrombocytopenic purpura. Blood 2010;116:4060–4069.
40 Bitzan M, Schaefer F, Reymond D: Treatment of typical (enteropathic) hemolytic uremic syndrome. Semin Thromb Hemost 2010;36:594–610.
41 Loirat C, Freemeaux-Bacchi V: Atypical hemolytic uremic syndrome. Orphanet J Rare Dis 2011;6:60.
42 Valent P, Klion AD, Horny HP, Roufosse F, Gotlib J, Weller PF, et al: Contemporary consensus proposal on criteria and classification of eosinophilic disorders and related syndromes. J Allergy Clin Immunol 2012;130:607–612.e9.
43 Gotlib J: World Health Organization-defined eosinophilic disorders: 2012 update on diagnosis, risk stratification, and management. Am J Hematol 2012; 87:903–914.
44 Jordan MB, Allen CE, Weitzman S, Filipovich AH, McClain KL: How I treat hemophagocytic lymphohistiocytosis. Blood 2011;118:4041–4052.
45 Gupta S, Weitzman S: Primary and secondary hemophagocytic lymphohistiocytosis: clinical features, pathogenesis and therapy. Expert Rev Clin Immunol 2010;6:137–154.

Shoshana Revel-Vilk, MD, MSc
Department of Pediatric Hematology/Oncology
Hadassah Hebrew University Hospital
IL–91200 Jerusalem (Israel)
E-Mail shoshanav@hadassah.org.il

Thomas AE, Halsey C (eds): Controversies in Pediatric and Adolescent Hematology.
Pediatr Adolesc Med. Basel, Karger, 2014, vol 17, pp 67–80 (DOI: 10.1159/000350347)

New Advances in the Treatment of Children with Hemophilia

David Lillicrap

Department of Pathology and Molecular Medicine, Richardson Laboratory, Queen's University, Kingston, Ont., Canada

Abstract

Current treatments for hemophilia are safe and effective, but during the past five years we have witnessed the development of a variety of novel therapies that are now beginning to enter the clinic. Evidence over an extended period from Scandinavia and more recent prospective randomized trial data have indicated that prophylactic strategies for factor replacement provide long-term musculoskeletal benefit in children with hemophilia. While the details of when factor prophylaxis should be initiated, and what prophylaxis protocol should be chosen are still matters of debate, recent innovations in hemophilia therapies are all aimed at facilitating prophylactic treatment. In general, efforts have been focused principally on developing replacement proteins with extended half-lives, although there have also been additional more early stage efforts to reduce factor VIII immunogenicity and enhance the coagulant activity of certain clotting factors. In the next 2–3 years, we will begin to see the introduction of several new clotting factor concentrates with increased half-lives. How these products will be used and how significant the uptake of these products will be remain to be seen. Finally, the recent first demonstration of clinical success of gene transfer for hemophilia suggests that this new treatment paradigm may also be a consideration for children with this condition at some point in the future.
Copyright © 2014 S. Karger AG, Basel

Current Treatment Approaches for Treatment of Hemophilia in Children

The two strategies for clotting factor replacement used in clinical practice are so-called on-demand treatments in which clotting factor replacement is given as early after a bleeding event as possible, and prophylactic therapy, in which concentrate is given on a regular basis to prevent bleeding. Experience with prophylactic treatment over several decades in Scandinavia has demonstrated the long-term musculoskeletal benefits of this mode of therapy [1] and, more recently, a randomized prospective study has confirmed these findings [2]. Thus, in countries in which access to clotting factor concentrates is not significantly constrained by economic influences, there has been a growing trend for starting prophylactic therapy early in childhood. The optimal time to start prophylaxis and the most effective/efficient prophylactic regimen remain matters of debate, but there is no doubt that the benefits for musculoskeletal health at least into early adulthood are significant with this treatment approach. Whether prophylaxis should be continued in all adults and what schedule of prophylaxis should be used is also unclear.

Clotting factor replacement currently utilizes plasma-derived and recombinant concentrates, with the choice of concentrate usually dependent upon financial considerations [3]. All clotting factor concentrates undergo viral inactivation processes, and there has now been an extended period since viral transmission was documented with these products. Thus, although there is still a theoretical risk of infectious agent transmission with clotting factor concentrates this can now be considered as an essentially historical complication. The transmissible spongiform encephalopathies represent a fortunately very rare exception to this rule, and measures to guard against the transmission of prions have now been instituted in the United Kingdom for an extended period of time. The major ongoing complication of clotting factor treatment is the development of inhibitory antibodies directed against the infused proteins. This complication occurs in approximately 25% of severe hemophilia A patients and develops after an average of 10–20 concentrate infusions; thus most often within the first 2–3 years of life [4]. In hemophilia B, the incidence of factor IX inhibitors is approximately 3% but in these patients the co-existence of anaphylaxis further complicates the clinical management [5]. The question of whether recombinant clotting factor concentrates, and particularly FVIII concentrates, are more immunogenic than their plasma-derived counterparts continues to provoke debate and is the subject of several ongoing prospective studies.

Limitations to Current Treatment Protocols for Hemophilia in Children

As discussed above, the major treatment-related complication of clotting factor concentrate use in hemophilia is the development of neutralizing antibodies in approximately 25% and 3% of severe hemophilia A and B patients, respectively. Aside from this complication, the major limitations to current replacement therapy are the inconvenience of intravenous infusion, rare allergic responses and the high cost of concentrates that restricts access to these products to less than 40% of the world's hemophilia population.

Strategies for Enhanced Therapy of Hemophilia in Children

In general, efforts to improve treatment approaches for hemophilia can be grouped into three categories: strategies to enhance the circulation time of clotting factors, initiatives to develop FVIII concentrates with reduced immunogenicity, and efforts to

- Clotting factors with prolonged half-lives
- Clotting factors with reduced immunogenicity
- Clotting factors with enhanced coagulant activity
- Intrinsic tenase complex substitutes
- Inhibition of natural anticoagulant pathways

Fig. 1. Potential approaches for the enhancement of hemophilia management in children.

generate replacement factors with enhanced specific coagulant activity (fig. 1). Suffice it to say that progress with the generation of FVIII proteins demonstrating reduced immunogenicity is still in an early stage of development and, given the complex nature of the anti-FVIII immune response, may prove challenging to translate into clinical practice. Similarly, with one or two exceptions [6], the development of hyperactive replacement molecules is of minor relevance for incorporation into clinical care in the near future. Thus, most new initiatives close to clinical application, or already in clinical trials, have addressed alternate modes of delivery or strategies for prolonging the half-life of the replacement proteins.

The necessity for intravenous administration of coagulation factor concentrates combined with the unequivocal demonstration that prophylactic schedules of treatment result in enhanced long-term musculoskeletal outcomes has focused attention on the potential for alternate routes of concentrate delivery and on the development of products that require less frequent intravenous administration. An oral clotting factor preparation would be the perfect solution to the challenges of intravenous administration in young children, but the physicochemical properties of FVIII and FIX suggest that this goal is highly unlikely to be attainable without a major advance in drug delivery science. Similarly, while some progress has been made with the formulation of products for subcutaneous administration, the high protein concentrations required for successful delivery via this route may also prove prohibitive.

Strategies for Enhancing the Half-Life of Clotting Factors

With average half-lives of 12 and 24 h, respectively, and even shorter half-lives in children, FVIII and FIX have to be administered 2–3 times each week to maintain adequate trough plasma levels to prevent spontaneous bleeding events. There is general consensus that the development of replacement therapies that would need to be administered just once a week, or even less often, would represent a significant advance for clinical care. Certainly in very young children with hemophilia, where venous access is a significant challenge, this advance would be highly beneficial.

In general, there are two potential approaches to extending the half-life of circulating clotting factors: modification of the clotting factor protein or sustained delivery

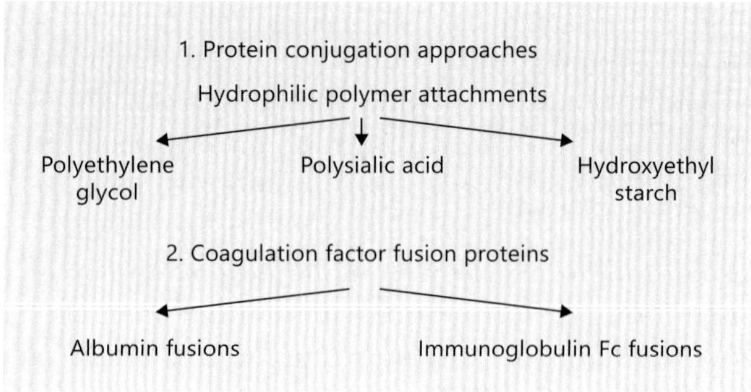

Fig. 2. Strategies for the development of therapeutic clotting factor products with prolonged half-lives.

of the protein through gene therapy. This review will discuss the relative merits of both strategies and their current status with regards to clinical application in children with hemophilia.

Modified Coagulation Factor Proteins with Prolonged Half-Lives

There are two major technologies that are now being used to modify the native FVIII and FIX proteins to enhance their circulating life spans. Currently, these strategies include the following: chemical modification with hydrophilic polymers and the generation of clotting factor fusion proteins (fig. 2).

Chemically Modified Clotting Factor Proteins

The principle of conjugating therapeutic proteins with hydrophilic polymers such as polyethylene glycol (PEG) has now been established for several decades. To date, several polymeric conjugates have been evaluated for use in modifying the half-life of clotting factors: most experience has been gained with PEG, but additional studies involving polysialic acid and hydroxyethyl starch have also been undertaken. A noteworthy difference between these last two polymers and PEG is that polysialic acid and hydroxyethyl starch are biodegradable, while in contrast, there is no natural removal pathway for PEG.

The chemical nature of these modifying polymers is diverse and complex, and thus markedly different outcomes can be obtained depending upon the size and structure of the chosen polymer. In addition, the mechanism of conjugation is also variable. Thus conjugation can be random in nature with multiple different sites in the partner molecule being modified or the modification can be targeted to one or several specific residues in the clotting factor sequence. For modification of FVIII and FIX the latter, targeted approach to polymer conjugation has become the preferred bioengineering strategy [7, 8]. This approach has the advantage of generating a homogeneous product with predictable activity in the clotting cascade intrinsic tenase complex, in which FVIII and FIX play key roles as cofactor and enzyme respectively (see below). In some instances, the conjugation involves attachment to specific amino acid residues and in other cases to carbohydrate.

The rationale for employing polymer conjugation strategies is 2-fold: first it is hoped that the hydrophilic 'shield' represented by the attached polymer reduces the interaction of the clotting factor protein with its clearance receptors; second, and of potential additional advantage, the polymer 'shield' might also minimize the interaction of the clotting factor protein with cells of the host immune system and thus reduce the risk for subsequent inhibitor development. While this latter capability has been demonstrated in vitro and in animal models, there is also evidence that polymer conjugation can sometimes enhance immunogenicity. Therefore, the potential immunogenicity of individual conjugated proteins must be assessed independently. The other potential limitation of these polymer conjugation protocols is the possibility of adversely interfering with the protein interactions in the intrinsic tenase complex, the assembly of FIXa (enzyme), FVIIIa (cofactor) and FX (substrate) on a phospholipid surface to generate FXa (product). Thus excessive polymer shielding or polymer attachments in certain locations may sterically hinder the crucial alignment of the enzyme-cofactor-substrate complex on activated phospholipid surfaces and reduce catalytic efficiency to unacceptable levels.

Results of Clotting Factor Conjugation Strategies

To date, the only polymer that has been evaluated in this context has been PEG, with different linkage technologies being employed by different biopharmaceutical companies. A strategy of glycoPEGylation (on posttranslationally added glycans) has been used for both FVIII and FIX [8], while targeted PEG conjugation to specific amino acid residues has been utilized in modifying FVIII [7].

The results of currently available preclinical and early-phase clinical studies with these conjugated concentrates have shown gratifyingly consistent outcomes with half-life extensions for FIX of 3- to 5-fold and for FVIII of 1.5- to 2-fold. These results indicate that prophylactic infusions of FIX to maintain trough levels protective against spontaneous bleeding will only need to be administered once a week, or in some patients even less frequently. Clearly, and especially in the case of young children, this advance will be of considerable practical benefit and one envisages widespread switching to these new FIX concentrates once they have received regulatory approval. In contrast, the increment in half-life for FVIII, while still significant, is not as dramatic and will likely result in a more individualized approach to choosing concentrates. However, in young children with challenging venous access, even a 1.5- to 2-fold half-life extension may be reason enough to switch to using these new concentrates.

As can be seen below, in the text relating to clotting factor fusion protein generation, very similar half-life extensions appear to be achievable for FVIII and FIX with any of these modifications. The obvious question posed by these findings is therefore why is there such a big difference between the influence on FIX and FVIII? Before attempting to answer this question, it is worthwhile highlighting the fact that our basic knowledge of the mechanisms involved in the clearance of FVIII and FIX is very limited. Cells in the liver and spleen appear to be involved in this process, but aside from a role for low-density lipoprotein receptor-related protein 1 (LRP-1) in clearing FVIII [9], very little else is known. Currently, the best explanation for the difference in the ability to modify FVIII and FIX half-lives is that FVIII clearance is dominantly influenced by its interaction with von Willebrand factor (VWF) and that the PEG modification of FVIII only partially overcomes the VWF effect. The half-life of FVIII in the absence of VWF is only 2 h, but in the presence of this carrier protein, it appears that extensions of half-life greater than those documented in the recent clinical trials of modified FVIII molecules will require further innovative strategies.

Issues for Future Consideration in the Clinical Utility of Molecular Conjugates in Hemophilia

Studies to date have shown good in vitro and in vivo hemostatic efficacy of these conjugates with no demonstrable adverse effects. As with all hemostatic therapies, there will be a requirement for these treatments to be monitored with appropriate laboratory testing and the performance of these concentrates in functional FVIII and FIX assays will need to be carefully evaluated. In some instances, the performance of these assays may require the use of a product-specific standard.

While the prolongation of clotting factor half-lives appears consistent and significant for both FVIII and FIX there were initial concerns about the ability of these concentrates to provide immediate hemostatic efficacy at the time of an acute bleed or for surgical hemostasis. These concerns do not appear to be well founded and, aside from the fact the protein will be cleared more slowly and thus dosing schedules will need to be revised, there is no reason that these new products cannot be used for the treatment of bleeding.

As alluded to above, while some pharmacologically utilized polymers are biodegradable, PEG is not, and it appears that over time, PEG accumulates in phagocytic cells in the reticuloendothelial system. In children with hemophilia using these concentrates for prophylactic treatment over many years, this cumulative effect will of course be accentuated. Whether this accumulation of PEG in phagocytes adversely influences the host immune function in the long-term is unknown, and requires more detailed assessment in animal models.

The final issue that must be considered with all of the new clotting factor concentrates is the potential for enhanced immunogenicity. While there has been no suggestion of this complication in any of the preclinical and early-phase clinical studies, formal postmarketing surveillance programs will need to be developed to evaluate the possibility of neo-immunogenicity as a result of the structural changes made to the clotting factors.

Coagulation Factor Fusion Proteins

The second approach that has been used to extend the half-life of FVIII and FIX is the generation of fusion proteins with either albumin or the Fc region of immunoglobulin.

In both strategies, the fusion proteins are synthesized as recombinant proteins using fused cDNA sequences for the clotting factor and either human albumin or the Fc chain of immunoglobulin. In the albumin fusion constructs, a small (~30 amino acid) flexible linker region is included between the C-terminus of the clotting factor protein and the fusion partner, while in the available Fc fusions, the Fc protein is linked directly to the clotting factor without a linker. In both cases, there appears to be little or no loss of specific coagulant function for the fusion protein [10, 11].

The extension of half-life mediated by these two types of fusion protein has the same mechanistic basis. With both immunoglobulin Fc and albumin fusions, recycling of the protein has been shown to be mediated by the neonatal Fc receptor (FcRn) present in the early endosomes of endothelial cells [12]. This recycling mechanism is responsible for the long half-lives of serum albumin and the immunoglobulins (~25 days) and it is this same receptor-mediated process that extends the half-lives of the FVIII and FIX fusions. Of significant interest, FcRn is also responsible for facilitating the transplacental movement of maternal immunoglobulins to the fetus [12]. This suggests that a similar mechanism might act to transfer the FVIII and FIX Fc fusion to hemophilic fetuses, a function that could have positive implications for both attaining central immunological tolerance to the clotting factors, and also possibly for developing effective hemostasis at the time of delivery. These potential outcomes require appropriate initial evaluation in animal models of hemophilia.

Results of Clotting Factor Fusion Protein Development

Perhaps, somewhat surprisingly, given that the mechanism of half-life extension is so different, the results obtained with these products have been very similar to those documented with the molecular conjugates, that is, FVIII half-life extensions of 1.5- to 2-fold and FIX half-life prolongations of 3- to 5-fold [11, 13, 14]. Why these outcomes are so similar is unclear, but again, with so little knowledge about normal clearance processes for the native proteins, this question is very difficult to address.

As with the FVIII and FIX conjugates, the preclinical and early-phase clinical studies of these fusion concentrates have been characterized by excellent hemostasis and a lack of significant adverse events including the appearance of inhibitory antibodies.

These novel fusion proteins are, like the FVIII and FIX conjugates, ideally suited for use in prophylaxis schedules of hemophilia treatment. The marked extension of half-life with the FIX fusions and the resulting reduction of concentrate administration to once weekly (or even less frequently) makes the incorporation of these products into hemophilia clinical care appear highly desirable. The uptake of the FVIII fusions will likely be more circumspect, but again in children where venous access is so crucial, they may also find increasing use. Once again, it should be emphasized that these extended half-life fusion proteins also have excellent acute hemostatic efficacy and can thus be used to good effect for treating bleeding episodes and for effecting surgical hemostasis.

Issues for Future Consideration in the Clinical Utility of Clotting Factor Fusion Proteins in Hemophilia

The caveats that need to be contemplated for the clotting factor fusion proteins are identical to those detailed for the molecular conjugates with the exception that the fusions will be cleared and degraded without any cumulative effects.

There has been no evidence of enhanced immunogenicity in the reported pre-clinical and early phase clinical studies and given that all of the protein sequences aside from the fusion junctions and linker regions are native structures, such enhanced immune reactivity is not expected.

Finally, as with the conjugated concentrates, attention will need to be paid to the performance of these products in clinical clotting assays, and in particular, in one-stage FVIII and FIX assays. Whether product-specific standards will be required to evaluate post-infusion plasma levels of these proteins is not yet clear.

Choosing Extended Half-Life Clotting Factor Concentrates for Children with Hemophilia

The successful development of several FVIII and FIX proteins with prolonged half-lives will begin to impact the care of children with hemophilia in the very near future. It is anticipated that some of these products will receive regulatory approval in the next 1–2 years and will be available for widespread clinical use.

The FIX extended half-life products offer major advantages in terms of a reduction in the frequency of administration and switching children with severe hemophilia B to these products for prophylactic therapy is an obvious choice. The decision of whether to use a FIX conjugate or fusion protein is far less easy and should involve a detailed discussion of the product attributes with the child and family. The only clear difference between the two forms of therapy, the accumulation of PEG over time, is of uncertain significance at this time. Although the initial reports of FIX half-life extension for these various products have shown some differences, it remains to be seen whether these differences are significant in clinical practice.

As discussed above, switching children to the new extended half-life FVIII products may not be such an easy choice, given the more modest, although significant extensions to survival of the new proteins. Patient-specific decisions concerning product switches will need to be made following consultation with the patient and his (or her) family.

Enhancements and Substitutions to the Intrinsic Tenase Complex

While hemophilia treatment protocols have relied upon protein replacement approaches for the past 50 years, there may now be the potential for novel strategies to reconstitute a functional intrinsic tenase complex in the absence of normal FVIII or FIX.

The first approach that has been evaluated is the development of hyperactive FIX molecules that have the capability of generating some FXa in the absence of FVIIIa. This concept has been tested in both hemophilia A and B mice and has been shown to produce physiologically relevant levels of hemostasis [6]. However, this strategy is still a long way from clinical translation, and the major concern, that of an acquired hypercoagulable state, still remains to be evaluated.

The second strategy that has attracted attention is the development of molecules that can substitute for the hemostatic cofactor activity of FVIIIa, so-called FVIII mimetics. Although the precise co-factor function of FVIIIa remains unclear, it appears to act as a structural scaffold on which enzyme (FIXa) and substrate (FX) are optimally aligned on a phospholipid surface (the activated platelet membrane). Attempts to mimic this role have been pursued for some time and agents such as bispecific antibodies (binding FIXa and FX) have been developed [15]. Whether the precise and controlled function of FVIIIa can indeed be replicated with a synthetic mimetic remains to be seen, but the successful development of such a molecule would be a transformative technology in terms of future hemophilia management.

Innovative Adjunctive Therapies for Hemophilia in Children

Adjunctive agents are already in use for hemophilia management in the form of antifibrinolytic therapies (tranexamic acid and epsilon-caproic acid) that are often administered together with clotting factor concentrates for dental and surgical procedures and some types of spontaneous bleeding. This management approach suggests that for most bleeding situations some form of replacement/substitution of the proteins involved in the intrinsic tenase complex assembly will be required to achieve adequate hemostasis. This observation presumably emphasizes the crucial physiological role of the amplification/propagation phase of the hemostatic process.

Recently, a number of efforts have been made to develop novel adjunctive pro-hemostatic agents that involve interference with normal anticoagulant processes. Most work has focused on the inhibition of the tissue factor pathway inhibitor (TFPI). There are now a variety of antibody, peptide and nucleic acid-mediated (DNA aptamers and siRNA) strategies to reduce TFPI activity that are undergoing preclinical and early-phase clinical assessment [16, 17]. The in vivo efficacy of these approaches and the resulting enhancement of thrombin generation and ultimately fibrin formation has been documented in preclinical models for some of these methodologies but further phase I/II studies are awaited with interest. In addition to the inhibition of TFPI, there is also interest in 'knocking down' other anticoagulant proteins including protein C, protein S and antithrombin. These early stage investigations are again using a variety of antibody and nucleic acid-based approaches. In all of these approaches, it seems likely that coincident intrinsic tenase reconstitution will be required to achieve therapeutically relevant hemostasis. Finally, if the strategy of inhibiting anticoagulant proteins as an adjunctive therapy for hemophilia reaches the clinic, the issue of potential thrombogenicity will need to be kept in mind. At the least, patients will need to be screened for pre-existing thrombophilic traits prior to the initiation of these therapies.

Not all of these adjunctive strategies have involved protein synthetic or bioengineering technologies. Interestingly, the natural sulfated polysaccharide, fucoidan, derived from brown algae, has been shown to possess significant pro-coagulant effects, mediated at least in part through an anti-TFPI effect. In the dog model of hemophilia A, the pro-hemostatic effect of fucoidan was dose-dependent, and at higher doses showed a major improvement in thromboelastometry tracings [18]. Furthermore, the particular formulation of the material used in these experiments had good bioavailability when administered by both subcutaneous and oral routes. However, the chemical composition of fucoidan is complex and very heterogeneous (not unlike its chemical relative, unfractionated heparin), and until a fractionated product that retains the pro-coagulant properties of the native material is available so that quality and consistency of the product can be assured, the therapeutic potential of this compound remains unclear.

The final comment that merits inclusion in this discussion of these adjunctive agents relates to laboratory monitoring. None of these agents will be evaluable with routine tests of clotting (e.g. PT, APTT, thrombin time or single factor assays) and thus some form of global hemostatic test will be required to assess their clinical benefit. The two tests that are leading candidates for the reproducible evaluation of global hemostasis are the thrombin generation assay and thromboelastography [19, 20]. Suffice it to say that while both of these tests have shown significant potential in the research setting, and in occasional clinical contexts, the standardization of both types of assay remains a significant challenge, and it is unlikely that they will enter widespread clinical application in the near future.

Novel Hemostatic Bypass Products

The development of neutralizing antibodies to FVIII occur in approximately 25% of patients with severe hemophilia and this complication usually occurs in the first few years of life after 10–20 exposures to FVIII concentrates.

In these children, FVIII replacement is ineffective and thus, some form of hemostatic bypass agent is required to treat or prevent bleeding. Currently, the two bypass products in clinical practice are recombinant factor VIIa (rFVIIa) and FEIBA (factor eight inhibitor bypass activity). Clinical trials have shown that these products have equivalent hemostatic efficacy in the treatment of bleeding in inhibitor patients with success rates of ~85% [21]. Both products are very expensive, and while the administration of both products is inconvenient, the 2- to 3-hour half-life of rFVIIa is a major limitation of this product.

Recently, steps have been taken to enhance the therapeutic convenience and efficacy of rFVIIa. Molecular conjugates and albumin fusions of rFVIIa have been developed that have shown considerable extensions of the protein's half-life [22]. In addition, other substitutions to the rFVIIa molecule have been made to accelerate its catalytic activity and enhance binding to phospholipid surfaces [23]. Early phase trials of some of these molecules are now underway.

Finally, after a prolonged absence from the clinic of porcine FVIII, a new recombinant product is now in early phase clinical trials. If finally approved, and in children whose anti-FVIII antibody is non-cross-reactive with the porcine protein, this heterologous form of FVIII could be a treatment alternative in children with inhibitors.

Gene Therapy for Children with Hemophilia

As classical monogenic, recessive X-linked disorders, the hemophilias have always been prime targets for the application of somatic cell gene transfer (gene therapy). While many pre-clinical studies of both FVIII and FIX gene transfer have proved successful over the past decade, it has not been until the past 2 years that we have witnessed evidence in human hemophilia of sustained expression of a clotting factor protein at therapeutically useful levels (fig. 3).

In the study reported in the *New England Journal of Medicine* in December 2011, a FIX adeno-associated vector delivered by intravenous infusion to the liver showed significant long-term benefits in most of the six study participants [24]. Most importantly, in the 2 patients treated with the highest vector dose (2×10^{12} vector genomes/kg), plasma levels of FIX between 3 and 8% have persisted beyond a year after a single vector infusion. The only adverse event noted in 2 of these patients was a transient elevation of liver transaminases, almost certainly the result of cytotoxic T cell-mediated destruction of AAV transduced hepatocytes. The antigenic targets of

Hemophilia gene therapy: current status (August 2012)

- Recent success in 6 adults with severe hemophilia B
  - Transgene delivery with an AAV8 vector
  - 3–8% FIX levels maintained for >1 year
- No clinical successes as yet with FVIII gene therapy

Rationale for need to delay gene therapy in children with hemophilia

a) Loss of AAV vector as hepatocytes replicate with liver enlargement
b) Potential for long-term genotoxicity
c) Very good non gene-based alternative treatment strategies

Fig. 3. Current status of hemophilia gene therapy and reasons for the need to delay gene therapy trials in children with hemophilia.

these T cells appears to be AAV capsid sequences that are presented on the surface of transduced hepatocytes after vector uncoating and capsid degradation [25]. In each patient that experienced this event, a short course (4–6 weeks) of prednisone resulted in a return to normal of transaminase levels.

While these results are enormously encouraging after the 25-year wait to achieve clinical success with hemophilia gene therapy, there are many issues that require consideration and resolution before this therapeutic strategy could become 'mainstream'. This is especially the case for children with hemophilia. The recent AAV trial involved only adults, and there has been no consideration of applying this treatment strategy to children. The main limitation of using this approach in children is that the majority of AAV persists in transduced cells as extrachromosomal concatemers and, thus, with the replication of liver cells, as occurs with normal childhood development as the liver enlarges, the vector sequences are lost and the therapeutic effect is progressively diluted.

The other rationale for delaying the implementation of gene transfer in children with hemophilia is the potential long-term genotoxic adverse effects. While AAV, clearly the current lead candidate vector type for gene therapy of hemophilia, does not actively integrate into the host genome, the vector does get inserted at sites of natural breaks in chromosomes [26]. While the existing evidence from animal studies suggests that these insertion events are likely to be benign, until long-term follow-up (>10 years) of AAV-treated adults has been completed it would be ill-advised to initiate gene therapy studies in children.

Aside from the significant caveats raised above concerning gene therapy initiatives in children with hemophilia, it is also important to recognize that while successful protocols may now be feasible for adult hemophilia B subjects, the attainment of successful FVIII gene transfer has still not been possible. This goal may be challenged by a number of significant obstacles including vector packaging constraints, low levels of transgene expression and, finally, immune responses to both the vector and the transgene protein.

Thus, in conclusion, while hemophilia gene therapy may now be entering a new era of optimism, at least for adults with severe hemophilia B, the application of this therapeutic paradigm to children with hemophilia is still a distant possibility, unless there are transformative advances to methodologies such as nonviral gene transfer and in situ mutation repair.

Concluding Remarks

After a 50-year period in which hemophilia has been treated exclusively with clotting factor concentrate replacement, there is now a range of novel therapeutic strategies that are in late stage preclinical or early-stage clinical development. While the initial focus of these developments has been on prolonging the half-lives of these proteins, there are also initiatives to reduce immunogenicity, to establish alternate modes of factor delivery and even to create synthetic substitutes for components of the intrinsic tenase complex.

These are exciting times for the entire hemophilia scientific, clinical and patient communities. There is a very realistic hope that these therapeutic advances will result in significant improvements to the quality of life and long-term health of children with these conditions. The other important change that will accompany the arrival of these new therapies is that clinicians will need to be prepared to develop rational approaches to choosing which treatment is best for specific patients, rather than simply choosing a FVIII or FIX concentrate. This array of new therapeutic strategies reminds us once again of what an excellent model disease hemophilia is for the application of innovative molecular science.

References

1 Nilsson IM, Berntorp E, Lofqvist T, Pettersson H: Twenty-five years' experience of prophylactic treatment in severe haemophilia A and B. J Intern Med 1992;232:25–32.
2 Manco-Johnson MJ, Abshire TC, Shapiro AD, Riske B, Hacker MR, Kilcoyne R, Ingram JD, Manco-Johnson ML, Funk S, Jacobson L, Valentino LA, Hoots WK, Buchanan GR, DiMichele D, Recht M, Brown D, Leissinger C, Bleak S, Cohen A, Mathew P, Matsunaga A, Medeiros D, Nugent D, Thomas GA, Thompson AA, McRedmond K, Soucie JM, Austin H, Evatt BL: Prophylaxis versus episodic treatment to prevent joint disease in boys with severe hemophilia. N Engl J Med 2007;357:535–544.
3 Key NS, Negrier C: Coagulation factor concentrates: past, present, and future. Lancet 2007;370:439–448.
4 Hay CRM, Palmer B, Chalmers E, Liesner R, Maclean R, Rangarajan S, Williams M, Collins PW: Incidence of factor VIII inhibitors throughout life in severe hemophilia A in the United Kingdom. Blood 2011;117:6367–6370.
5 DiMichele D: Inhibitor development in haemophilia B: an orphan disease in need of attention. Br J Haematol 2007;138:305–315.
6 Schuettrumpf J, Herzog RW, Schlachterman A, Kaufhold A, Stafford DW, Arruda VR: Factor IX variants improve gene therapy efficacy for hemophilia B. Blood 2005;105:2316–2323.
7 Mei B, Pan C, Jiang H, Tjandra H, Strauss J, Chen Y, Liu T, Zhang X, Severs J, Newgren J, Chen J, Gu JM, Subramanyam B, Fournel MA, Pierce GF, Murphy JE: Rational design of a fully active, long-acting PEGylated factor VIII for hemophilia A treatment. Blood 2010;116:309–315.

8 Negrier C, Knobe K, Tiede A, Giangrande P, Møss J: Enhanced pharmacokinetic properties of a glycoPEGylated recombinant factor IX: a first human dose trial in patients with hemophilia B. Blood 2011;118:2695–2701.
9 Schwarz HP, Lenting PJ, Binder B, Mihaly J, Denis C, Dorner F, Turecek PL: Involvement of low-density lipoprotein receptor-related protein (LRP) in the clearance of factor VIII in von Willebrand factor-deficient mice. Blood 2000;95:1703–1708.
10 Peters RT, Low SC, Kamphaus GD, Dumont JA, Amari JV, Lu Q, Zarbis-Papastoitsis G, Reidy TJ, Merricks EP, Nichols TC, Bitonti AJ: Prolonged activity of factor IX as a monomeric Fc fusion protein. Blood 2010;115:2057–2064.
11 Santagostino E, Negrier C, Klamroth R, Tiede A, Pabinger-Fasching I, Voigt C, Jacobs I, Morfini M: Safety and pharmacokinetics of a novel recombinant fusion protein linking coagulation factor IX with albumin (rIX-FP) in hemophilia B patients. Blood 2012;120:2405–2411.
12 Kuo TT, Baker K, Yoshida M, Qiao S-W, Aveson VG, Lencer WI, Blumberg RS: Neonatal Fc receptor: from immunity to therapeutics. J Clin Immunol 2010;30:777–789.
13 Shapiro AD, Ragni MV, Valentino LA, Key NS, Josephson NC, Powell JS, Cheng G, Thompson AR, Goyal J, Tubridy KL, Peters RT, Dumont JA, Euwart D, Li L, Hallén B, Gozzi P, Bitonti AJ, Jiang H, Luk A, Pierce GF: Recombinant factor IX-Fc fusion protein (rFIXFc) demonstrates safety and prolonged activity in a phase 1/2a study in hemophilia B patients. Blood 2012;119:666–672.
14 Powell JS, Josephson NC, Quon D, Ragni MV, Cheng G, Li E, Jiang H, Li L, Dumont JA, Goyal J, Zhang X, Sommer J, McCue J, Barbetti M, Luk A, Pierce GF: Safety and prolonged activity of recombinant factor VIII Fc fusion protein in hemophilia A patients. Blood 2012;119:3031–3037.
15 Takeyama M, Nogami K, Matsumoto T, Soeda T, Suzuki T, Hattori K, Shima M: Characterisation of an antibody specific for coagulation factor VIII that enhances factor VIII activity. Thromb Haemost 2010;103:94–102.
16 Gorczyca ME, Nair SC, Jilma B, Priya S, Male C, Reitter S, Knoebl P, Gilbert JC, Schaub RG, Dockal M, McGinness KE, Pabinger I, Srivastava A: Inhibition of tissue factor pathway inhibitor by the aptamer BAX499 improves clotting of hemophilic blood and plasma. J Thromb Haemost 2012;10:1581–1590.
17 Hilden I, Lauritzen B, Sørensen BB, Clausen JT, Jespersgaard C, Krogh BO, Bowler AN, Breinholt J, Gruhler A, Svensson LA, Petersen HH, Petersen LC, Balling KW, Hansen L, Hermit MB, Egebjerg T, Friederichsen B, Ezban M, Bjørn SE: Hemostatic effect of a monoclonal antibody mAb 2021 blocking the interaction between FXa and TFPI in a rabbit hemophilia model. Blood 2012;119:5871–5878.
18 Prasad S, Lillicrap D, Labelle A, Knappe S, Keller T, Burnett E, Powell S, Johnson KW: Efficacy and safety of a new-class hemostatic drug candidate, AV513, in dogs with hemophilia A. Blood 2008;111:672–679.
19 van Geffen M, van Heerde WL: Global haemostasis assays, from bench to bedside. Thromb Res 2012;129:681–687.
20 Chitlur M: Challenges in the laboratory analyses of bleeding disorders. Thromb Res 2012;130:1–6.
21 Astermark J, Donfield SM, DiMichele DM, Gringeri A, Gilbert SA, Waters J, Berntorp E: A randomized comparison of bypassing agents in hemophilia complicated by an inhibitor: the FEIBA NovoSeven Comparative (FENOC) Study. Blood 2007;109:546–551.
22 Møss J, Rosholm A, Laurén A: Safety and pharmacokinetics of a glycoPEGylated recombinant activated factor VII derivative: a randomized first human dose trial in healthy subjects. J Thromb Haemost 2011;9:1368–1374.
23 Gray LD, Hussey MA, Larson BM, Machlus KR, Campbell RA, Koch G, Ezban M, Hedner U, Wolberg AS: Recombinant factor VIIa analog NN1731 (V158D/E296V/M298Q-FVIIa) enhances fibrin formation, structure and stability in lipidated hemophilic plasma. Thromb Res 2011;128:570–576.
24 Nathwani AC, Tuddenham EGD, Rangarajan S, Rosales C, McIntosh J, Linch DC, Chowdary P, Riddell A, Pie AJ, Harrington C, O'Beirne J, Smith K, Pasi J, Glader B, Rustagi P, Ng CYC, Kay MA, Zhou J, Spence Y, Morton CL, Allay J, Coleman J, Sleep S, Cunningham JM, Srivastava D, Basner-Tschakarjan E, Mingozzi F, High KA, Gray JT, Reiss UM, Nienhuis AW, Davidoff AM: Adenovirus-associated virus vector-mediated gene transfer in hemophilia B. N Engl J Med 2011;365:2357–2365.
25 Mingozzi F, High KA: Immune responses to AAV in clinical trials. Curr Gen Ther 2011;11:321–330.
26 Li H, Malani N, Hamilton SR, Schlachterman A, Bussadori G, Edmonson SE, Shah R, Arruda VR, Mingozzi F, Wright JF, Bushman FD, High KA: Assessing the potential for AAV vector genotoxicity in a murine model. Blood 2011;117:3311–3319.

Dr. David Lillicrap
Department of Pathology and Molecular Medicine
Richardson Laboratory, Queen's University
Kingston, ONT K7L 3N6 (Canada)
E-Mail lillicrap@cliff.path.queensu.ca

Thomas AE, Halsey C (eds): Controversies in Pediatric and Adolescent Hematology.
Pediatr Adolesc Med. Basel, Karger, 2014, vol 17, pp 81–97 (DOI: 10.1159/000350348)

Myelodysplastic and Myeloproliferative Diseases in Children: Current Concepts

Paresh Vyas

Department of Haematology and MRC Molecular Haematology Unit, Haematology and Cancer Centre, Weatherall Institute of Molecular Medicine, Oxford University Hospitals and Oxford University, Oxford, UK

Abstract

Paediatric myelodysplasia syndromes (MDS) and myeloproliferative disorders (MPD) are rare and genetically and clinically heterogeneous. This review focuses on recent studies outlining the partially characterised pathogenetic germline and/or acquired genetic changes in these disorders, how these changes perturb haemopoiesis and the implications for clinical practice. Identification of causative genetic changes in paediatric MDS/MPD will gather pace as genomes of these disorders are sequenced. These genetic findings are likely to provide a clearer definition of clinically and biologically distinct entities and improve classification of these disorders. Analysis of genetic changes in sequential samples as a disease progresses will allow an understanding of how acquisition of genetic changes during clinical follow-up may mark different clinical courses. Finally, studying the function of the altered proteins resulting from genetic change will hopefully lead to a deeper understanding of the cellular and molecular basis of these disorders with the potential to improve clinical management. Within paediatric MDS/MPD, entities such as juvenile myelomonocytic leukemia and myeloid disorders in Down syndrome are better defined, whereas others, such as sporadic myelodysplasia and essential thrombocytosis and primary polycythaemia have been more difficult to study because of their rarity and clinical and genetic heterogeneity. This review will not cover Philadelphia-positive chronic myeloid leukaemia.

Copyright © 2014 S. Karger AG, Basel

Classification

The World Health Organization (WHO) classification of haematological malignancies (table 1) incorporates distinct paediatric myelodysplasia syndromes/myeloproliferative disorders (MDS/MPD) entities [1, 2].

Table 1. Classification of paediatric MDS and MPD

1	Down syndrome disease
	Transient abnormal myelopoiesis
	Myeloid leukaemia of Down syndrome
2	Philadelphia chromosome-negative *BCR-ABL1*- negative MDS/MPD
	Juvenile myelomonocytic leukaemia
	Chronic myelomonocytic leukaemia (secondary only)
	Philadelphia chromosome-negative *BCR-ABL1*-negative chronic myelogenous leukaemia (CML)
	Essential thrombocytosis (ET)
	Primary polycythaemia vera (PRV)
	Myelofibrosis
	Primary myelofibrosis
	Myelofibrosis secondary to ET or PRV or an antecedent haematological disorder
3	Myelodysplastic syndrome
	Refractory cytopenia of childhood (peripheral blood blasts <2% and bone marrow blasts <5%)
	Refractory anaemia with excess of blasts (RAEB) (peripheral blood blasts 2–19% or bone marrow blasts 5–19%)
	RAEB in transformation (peripheral blood blasts or bone marrow blasts 20–29%)

This paediatric approach allows unambiguous classification of more than 95% of patients (for a review, see [3]). It includes juvenile myelomonocytic leukaemia (JMML) and myeloid disorders affecting children with Down syndrome (DS) as separate entities. Furthermore, paediatric MDS is subdivided differently from adult MDS. All refractory cytopenias without an excess of blasts are pooled into a single category of refractory cytopenia of childhood (RCC) (peripheral blood blast count <2% and bone marrow blasts <5%). In contrast to adult practice, the MDS subtypes 5q– syndrome and refractory anaemia with ring sideroblasts are virtually absent in paediatrics; furthermore, the significance of multilineage dysplasia in children is unknown. Refractory anaemia with an excess of blasts (RAEB) (peripheral blood blast count of 2–19% and/or bone marrow blasts 5–19%) was not subdivided into RAEB-I (bone marrow blasts 6–10%) and RAEB-II (bone marrow blasts 11–19%), as in adult practice. In paediatric practice, RAEB-T (peripheral blood and/or bone marrow blasts 20–29%) has been retained and a blast count of ≥30% has been required for a diagnosis of paediatric acute myeloid leukaemia (AML), as there are no data in children to indicate whether a blast threshold of 20% is better than 30% to distinguish MDS from AML. Patients who progress from MDS to AML may retain the biological characteristics of MDS and have been classified as MDS-related AML. However, given the difficulties in interobserver quantitation of a blast count and the biologic and clinical overlap between RAEB-T and AML, most clinicians understand that a comprehensive assessment of the tempo of the clinical and haematologic course coupled with an assessment of morphology, immunophenotype, and cytogenetics is required in the clinical management of any individual patient. Finally, in addition to these disease categories children can also rarely develop sporadic, non-familial essential thrombocytosis [4, 5], primary polycythaemia vera [6, 7] and primary and secondary myelofibrosis [8–11]. Though the definition of these disorders for children currently is the same as those for adult patients with these disorders, there are differences in clinical and genetic features between adults and children [7, 12].

Epidemiology

These are rare disorders. By identifying cases of MDS from population- and hospital-based registries the annual incidence of MDS and JMML has been estimated between 0.8 and 1.8 per million children aged 0–14 years in Denmark, Canada and the United Kingdom (see [3] for references to work in this section). In Japan, JMML constitutes ~7.7% of all paediatric leukaemias. Essential thrombocythaemia and polycythaemia vera are even rarer. With respect to MDS and JMML, the variation in incidence, in part, may reflect the different inclusion criteria used; for example, whether secondary MDS or disorders affecting newborns and children with DS are included. The male/female distribution in paediatric MDS is equal with a median age at presentation of 6.8 years.

Aetiology

Paediatric MDS/MPD disorders can either arise as familial or sporadic cases. In sporadic cases the causative genetic defects can arise either as de novo germline mutations or can be somatically acquired and be present only in blood cells. It is important to distinguish between these situations as it has implications for genetic counselling.

Primary MDS/MPD is defined as MDS/MPD that arises in a child with no antecedent haematological illness and who has not received therapy damaging to haematopoietic stem/progenitor cells. In primary MDS/MPD, it is assumed that the child either had silent germline genetic change(s) and/or acquired genetic change(s) without leading to an obvious disease phenotype.

MDS/MPD also arises in children who have had previous chemotherapy or radiotherapy therapy or an antecedent haematological disorder such as aplastic anaemia or bone marrow failure; in these cases, it is defined as secondary MDS/MPD.

Myeloid Disorders in Newborns and Children with Down Syndrome

Newborns and children with DS (trisomy 21, T21) below the age of 5 years are uniquely susceptible to two clonal myeloid disorders (reviewed in [13]):

(1) Transient abnormal myelopoiesis (TAM), also known as transient myeloproliferative disorder and transient leukaemia.

(2) Myeloid leukaemia of Down syndrome (ML-DS). Children with ML-DS often have an antecedent history of TAM. The two conditions are clonally linked and in most cases ML-DS is likely to have evolved from TAM (see below).

TAM – Clinical Findings

Though TAM is usually seen in newborns with DS, 7–16% of TAM cases have mosaic T21. TAM can also present as hydrops fetalis with hepatosplenomegaly. The current definition of TAM is imprecise. It is defined as the presence of circulating blood blasts in a baby with typical clinical features of TAM who may, or may not, have haematologic abnormalities. Previous studies have used differing clinical and/or haematologic criteria to define TAM [14–16]. At one end of the spectrum TAM is detected as an incidental finding on review of a blood smear in an otherwise well baby. Often there will be an associated mild leucocytosis and thrombocytopenia. At the other of the spectrum, babies can be extremely sick with bruising, ascites, jaundice, hepatosplenomegaly, respiratory distress associated with pleural effusions and a low cardiac output state associated with a pericardial effusion. In one series, 25% of the babies with TAM were referred to an intensive care unit [15].

TAM – Laboratory Findings

Laboratory tests can show leucocytosis (20–30% of cases with a mean white cell count of 20–40 × 10^9/l with occasional cases having a white count of >100 × 10^9/l) though it can be normal on occasion. There is variable thrombocytopenia in ~40% of cases (mean 80–100 × 10^9/l) and occasionally severe anaemia (haemoglobin <80 g/l). Basophilia and an eosinophilia are often seen. Blasts can have the appearance of megakaryoblasts (with cytoplasmic 'blebbing') but can also be featureless. Flow cytometry of blasts is helpful as they express CD34, CD38, CD117, CD7, CD56, CD33, CD45, the erythroid antigen CD235 and the megakaryocyte antigens CD41, CD42b and CD61. The bone marrow aspirate is not often helpful. The cellularity can be increased, normal or decreased. There is a deranged coagulation profile in 20–25% of cases with disseminated intravascular coagulation (DIC) in ~7–10% of cases. Hepatic dysfunction is usually associated with hyperbilirubinaemia, ascites, elevated transaminases and hepatic infiltration with blasts. In more severe cases, there is hepatic fibrosis. A diagnostic test in nearly all babies with TAM is the presence of acquired mutations within exon 2 and, occasionally, exon 3 of the gene encoding the key haematopoietic transcription factor *GATA1* (reviewed in [13]).

Outcome and Management of TAM

In most babies (80–90%) the condition only requires observation and blood count monitoring as it resolves spontaneously over a 1- to 3-month period (median time to resolution 47 days [16]). However, a proportion of babies require therapy for clinical symptoms, e.g. cardiac failure or DIC. However, it is unclear which infants will benefit from treatment and what the most effective treatment is. Accordingly treatment policies vary considerably between centres. Both the US Pediatric/Children's Oncology Group (POG/COG) and the German I-BFM group have developed treatment guidelines for TAM that can be instituted at the physician's discretion [15, 16].

As TAM blasts are highly sensitive to cytarabine, it is the basis of cytoreductive therapy. Response is generally rapid with disappearance of peripheral blasts within 7 days of treatment. However, in babies with severe liver disease associated with fibrosis the response to chemotherapy is poor. In the POG study 9481, cytosine arabinoside was given either as 10 or 1.2–1.5 mg/kg/dose subcutaneously or intravenously by slow injection twice a day for 7 days [14]. In the AML-BFM study, 0.5–1.5 mg/kg was administered for 3–12 days [15]. The higher dose of cytarabine (3.33 mg/kg/24 h given by continuous infusion for 5 days) used in the COG A2971 study is probably not required and was associated with significant toxicity [16].

Despite therapy, 10–20% of babies die of TAM within 3 months with hepatic and renal failure and DIC. These babies often present with a higher white count ($>100 \times 10^9$/l), ascites, effusions, coagulopathy and develop hepatic fibrosis.

Transformation to ML-DS

Some babies with a history of TAM develop ML-DS. The median age of onset of ML-DS is 1.4 years [14, 15]. Progression to ML-DS does not occur in children beyond the age of 5 years [17]. If AML develops in children with DS over age 5 it is usually AML of the type that can develop in any child and is not ML-DS.

Progression to ML-DS occurs at a variable tempo. In some children progression is heralded by a period of falling blood counts, especially thrombocytopenia and leucopenia. Cytopenia may be short or prolonged over months prior to formal diagnosis of ML-DS. It is often associated with dysplastic changes in peripheral blood cells. Rarely ML-DS can progress directly from aggressive TAM. In these cases the diagnosis is problematic as it is difficult to distinguish between TAM that is not resolving and development of ML-DS.

A bone marrow aspirate and trephine can be helpful to confirm >30% blasts. Often, the blast count is lower as the marrow sample on aspirate is haemodilute. In these cases, the trephine shows marrow fibrosis echoing the liver fibrosis seen in some cases of TAM. If the marrow is aspirable or if there are circulating blasts, flow cytometry is valuable as the blasts express the same cell-surface markers as TAM blasts. Once again, acquired *GATA1* mutations, of the type seen in TAM, are nearly always present and this provides a sensitive diagnostic test. In a baby with a history of TAM often the same *GATA1* mutation is detected when the child presents with ML-DS proving that the two disorders are clonally linked. In ~15–25% cases multiple *GATA1* mutations are detected in both TAM and ML-DS, suggesting that multiple GATA1 mutant clones exist [18].

Outcome of Treatment of ML-DS

For many years, children with DS received suboptimal treatment and had poor survival. However, as ML-DS is sensitive to cytosine arabinsoide, like TAM, there has been increasing recruitment to national leukaemia chemotherapy protocols. Contemporary regimens produce 5-year survival rates of 80% (see [19] for additional references). The main reason for treatment failure is toxicity (resistant disease and relapse are rare), predominantly due to mucositis and infection. Thus, current studies aim to reduce treatment intensity when compared with children with AML who do not have DS [20].

GATA1 Mutation, Definition of TAM and Silent TAM and Identification of Children at Risk of ML-DS

The incidence of TAM has been the subject of debate. Retrospective studies suggest that TAM affects ~10% of DS neonates but these studies have used differing clinical and/or hematologic criteria to define TAM, none of which is specific for TAM [14–16]. Importantly, no retrospective studies have systematically screened neonates for *GATA1* mutations, a genetic marker specific for TAM and ML-DS. Thus, current definitions of TAM neither specify the percentage of blasts considered abnormal in DS neonates nor the role of *GATA1* mutation analysis in the diagnosis. As a result, asymptomatic TAM may be missed in some neonates as blood counts and smears are often not performed. While in others babies, TAM may be overdiagnosed by relying on non-specific clinical and haematologic features. This possibility is borne out by the only large systematic *GATA1* mutation screen, performed by Sanger sequencing of genomic DNA extracted from dried blood spots, which found a prevalence of *GATA1* mutations in DS neonates of only 3.8% [21], in contrast to the 5–10% prevalence of TAM diagnosed by clinical and hematologic criteria (see review by [13]).

Thus, we embarked on a prospective study to systematically document clinical features, blood counts, blood smears and *GATA1* mutation in a large population-based cohort of newborns with DS. On evaluation of the first 200 babies all DS neonates had multiple blood count and smear abnormalities at birth. These included thrombocytopenia, polycythaemia, macrocytosis, and dysplastic change of all three myeloid lineages [Roberts et al., unpubl. data]. Surprisingly, 195/200 (97.5%) DS neonates had circulating blasts (range 1–77%). 17/200 (8.5%) DS neonates had *GATA1* mutations detected by conventional Sanger sequencing and/or denaturing high-performance liquid chromatography (DHPLC). In all cases where a *GATA1* mutation was detected by these techniques the blast count was >10%. To determine whether small mutant *GATA1* clones explain the frequent finding of blasts, we performed next-generation re-sequencing on 88 DS neonates without *GATA1* mutations detectable by conventional Sanger sequencing or DHPLC. Remarkably, 18/88 (20.4%) had small *GATA1* clones (sensitivity ~0.3%). All 18 had <10% blasts. No clinical or hematologic features distinguished them from *GATA1* mutation-negative DS neonates or cases of TAM. Thus, *GATA1* mutations are common, occur in ~28% of all neonates with DS but are

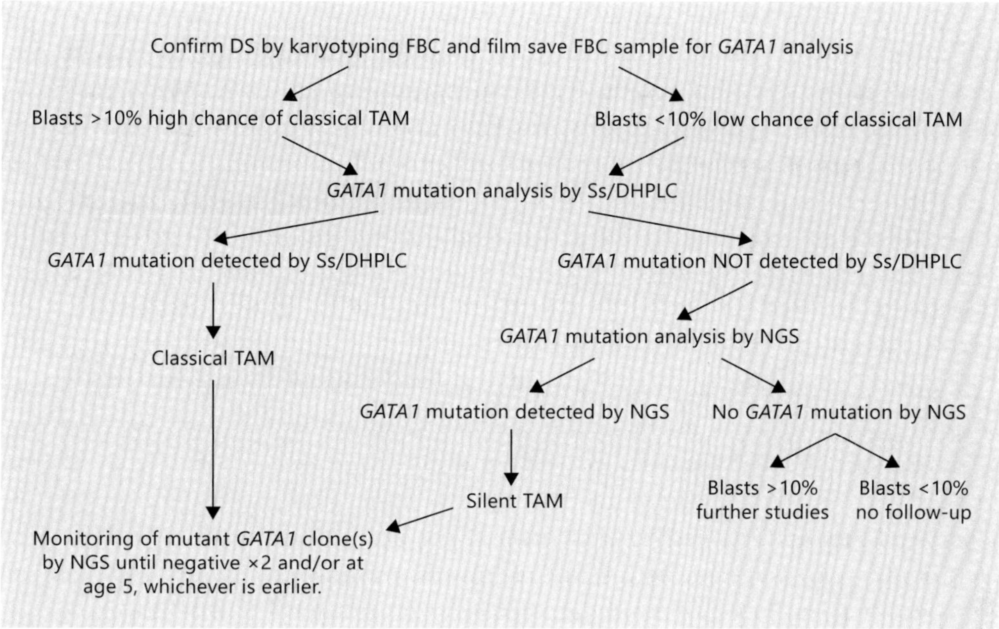

Fig. 1. Diagnosis and monitoring of mutant *GATA1* clones in DS. FBC = Full blood count; Ss = Sanger sequencing; DHPLC = denaturing high-performance liquid chromatography; NGS = next-generation re-sequencing.

often unsuspected and detectable only with sensitive methods. We suggest that TAM is defined as blasts >10% and a *GATA1* mutation detected by conventional sequencing and/or DHPLC. We suggest the term 'silent TAM' for those with a *GATA1* mutation detectable only by more sensitive sequencing techniques. In our series, both TAM and silent TAM can transform to ML-DS. Longer-term follow-up is required to determine rates of transformation. We favour a diagnostic algorithm (fig. 1) where evaluation of blood smears as well as full blood counts, as recommended by the American Academy of Pediatrics [22], is a useful, immediate screening step to identify DS neonates with 'classical' TAM who may require early treatment (especially where *GATA1* analysis is unavailable or delayed). We suggest all DS neonates should also have *GATA1* mutation analysis by Sanger sequencing and DHPLC to quickly identify those with large mutant *GATA1* clones. For DS neonates without mutations by Sanger sequencing or DHPLC, we suggest next generation re-sequencing is used to identify those with small mutant *GATA1* clones. By comprehensively detecting *GATA1* mutations, paediatric haematology follow-up can be limited to those at risk of transformation rather than all babies with blasts (i.e. ~all babies with DS).

Mechanisms of Oncogenesis in Myeloid Disorders of DS

Like many other childhood clonal disorders, including the acute leukaemias, the process for DS-associated leukaemia starts in fetal blood cells (see review by [13]).

The 'first hit' is T21, which expands fetal immunophenotypic haematopoietic stem cell compartment with erythroid-megakaryocyte biased differentiation leading to an expansion of megakaryocyte-erythroid progenitor [23]. The mechanisms by which T21 perturbs haematopoiesis are unclear and likely to be complex, involving not only a gene dosage effect of multiple genes on chromosome 21 but also indirectly through genes on other chromosomes. Plausible candidate genes on chromosome 21 with roles in megakaryocyte/erythroid differentiation or leukaemogenesis in ML-DS and TAM include *DRKYK1A*, *RUNX1, BACH1*, *ETS2* and *ERG* (see review by [23] for references). There are also 5 Hsa21 microRNAs, which may regulate haemopoiesis. Four of these are known to be expressed in human megakaryocyte lineage cells: miR-125b has been reported to be overexpressed in TAM and ML-DS in comparison with normal megakaryocytes; miR-99a expression increases during normal megakaryocyte differentiation while miR-155 and let-7c are expressed early in differentiation and decrease with megakaryocyte maturation. The identification and progressive refinement of the DS critical region (DSCR), which is estimated to cover a 4.3- to 5.4-Mb region of chromosome 21q22, has potentially reduced the number of candidate genes involved in DS leukaemogenesis, although the functional correlation between DSCR genes and clinical phenotype is still controversial.

T21 fetal blood stem cells then acquire *GATA1* mutations. Exome and whole genome sequencing of TAM and ML-DS and control samples show that *GATA1* mutation is the only consistent mutation required for TAM. Additional mutations in genes recurrently mutated in AML accompany transformation of TAM to ML-DS (see below).

GATA1 mutations produce an N-terminal truncated protein GATA1s or 'GATA1 short' protein. We now know from whole genome and exome sequencing that in most cases of TAM, only an acquired GATA1 mutation is required to develop TAM. Importantly, similar N-terminal *GATA1* mutations, in the absence of trisomy 21, cause cytopenia (including a Diamond-Blackfan phenotype) but not TAM or AML [24], underscoring the importance of cooperation between T21 and GATA1s protein in fetal blood stem/progenitor cells to cause the TAM phenotype.

The detailed mechanism(s) by which GATA1s promotes abnormal proliferation and differentiation of fetal, but not post-natal, megakaryocyte progenitors remain unclear [13]. Gene expression profiling suggests that changes in *GATA1*-mediated regulation of other transcription factors, including *GATA2, IKAROS, MYB* and *MYC*, are likely to be responsible for some of the functional effects of GATA1s expression in foetal megakaryocytes. It is also possible that there are significant effects due to loss of expression of full-length GATA1, such as impaired growth and differentiation of foetal/embryonic haematopoietic progenitors, which has been shown in a murine model. Recent studies show that GATA1s can transform fetal but not adult haematopoietic cells via overactivation of the insulin-like growth factor signalling pathway, suggesting that complex regulatory networks may be in play.

Whole genome and exome sequencing of TAM and ML-DS and control samples has shown that additional mutations accompany transformation of TAM to ML-DS. ML-DS samples had mean numbers of 5.8 non-synonymous mutations, i.e. mutations that are predicted to alter the sequence of the resulting protein per sample. Eight genes were recurrently mutated in ML-DS samples in whole exome sequencing, including *NRAS*, *TP53* and genes encoding components of the cohesin complex. Lower allelic burden of these additional mutations than corresponding *GATA1* mutations indicated that they were more likely to be subclonal mutations.

Juvenile Myelomonocytic Leukaemia

JMML is a rare but well-defined MPN that usually presents in infancy and young children and has an incidence of 1.2 cases per million (see review by [3] for references). JMML can occur either in an otherwise well infant/child or it can be part of a congenital syndrome. In either case the infant/child can present with fever, cough, bloody stools, with an accompanying intermittent erythematous rash, splenomegaly, persistent peripheral monocytosis of $>1 \times 10^9$/l and elevated haemoglobin F (50% of cases). The bone marrow is usually hypercellular with <20% blasts. Though monosomy 7 is seen in 25% of the cases, major advances in the identification of specific genetic mutations in JMML mean that now in 85–90% of children diagnostic germline or somatic mutations in the RAS/MAPK signalling pathway allow an unambiguous diagnosis to be made. Many of the advances in unravelling the genetics of JMML have come from the study of children with congenital syndromes who develop JMML including neurofibromatosis type 1 (see review by [25] for additional references) and its variants (e.g. Leopard's syndrome, Noonan's syndrome with multiple giant cell lesions, cardiac facio-syndrome and Costello's syndrome – reviewed in [26]) and germline CBL syndrome, i.e. patients with germline mutations in the proto-oncogene *CBL* which is a E3 ubiquitin protein ligase. The sum of a considerable amount of work has showed that sporadic or syndromal associated JMML arises from genetic mutations that lead to hyperactivation of the RAS/RAF/MEK/ERK signalling pathway (fig. 2).

What is clear is that molecular analysis is required to precisely define the molecular type of JMML and determine in the child if the mutation is somatic, de novo germline or inherited. This has implications not only for genetic counselling but also for an accurate clinical prognosis. As an example, patients with JMML in the context of Noonan's syndrome and homozygous *CBL* mutations have a high rate of spontaneous resolution of JMML, in a manner analogous to the resolution of DS-associated TAM. These subsets of JMML patients do not require definitive treatment such as allogeneic stem cell transplantation. Furthermore, rare children with homozygous *CBL* mutation, develop serious vasculopathies in the second decade of life [27]. Detailed discussion of the clinical management of JMML can be found elsewhere [25, 26].

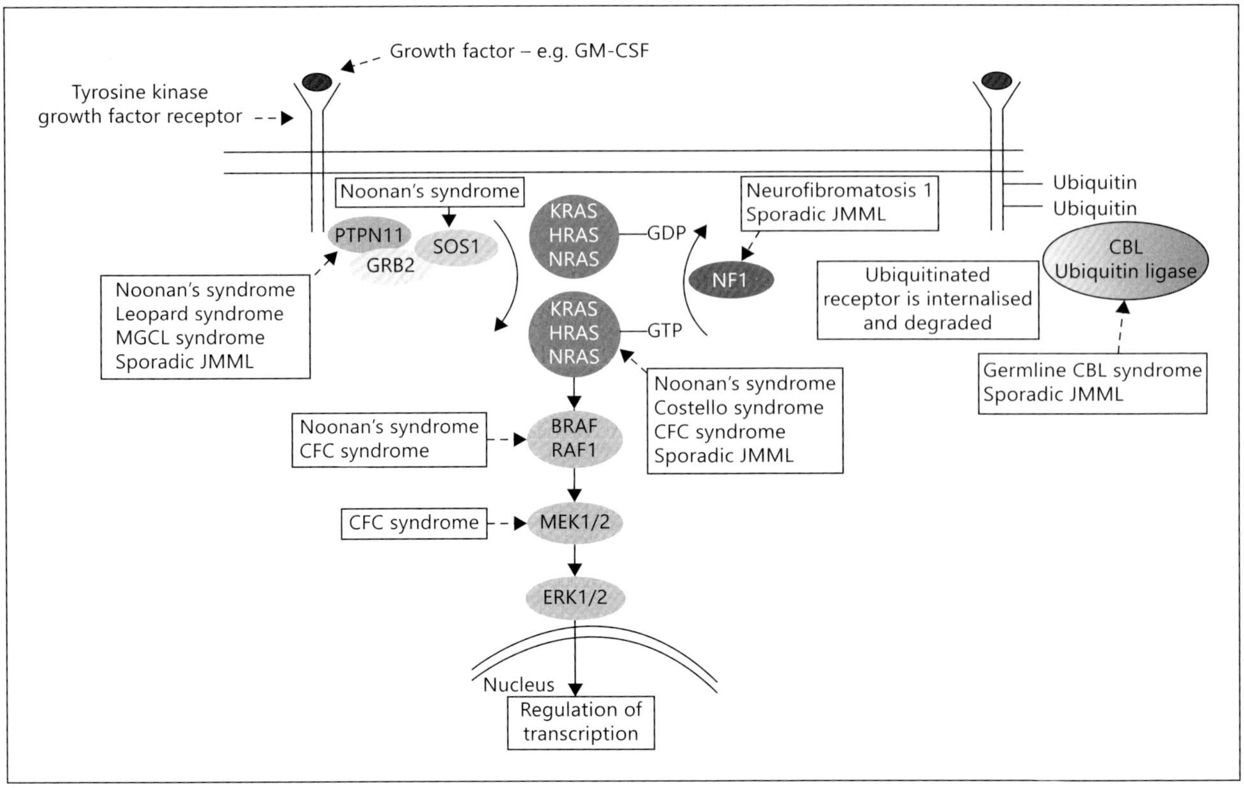

Fig. 2. Schematic diagram showing the RAS/RAF/MEK/ERK pathway and the location of mutations in syndromal and sporadic isolated JMML. CFC = Cardia-facio-cutaneous syndrome; MGCL = multiple giant cell lesion.

Secondary CMML

Secondary CMML is a rare diagnosis reserved for children with a prior history of chemotherapy or radiotherapy who develop persistent blood monocytosis $>1 \times 10^9$/l, and the absence of the Philadelphia chromosome, fewer than 20% blasts in peripheral blood or bone marrow, and an absence of eosinophilia and dysplasia in more than 1 lineage [1]. Data from retrospective series of therapy related paediatric MDS suggests this is rare even in the context of therapy-related paediatric MDS [28].

Philadelphia Chromosome-Negative Myeloproliferative Disorders

Philadelphia chromosome-negative *BCR-ABL1*-negative myeloproliferative neoplasms are very rare in children and this limits the data available to guide clinical practice. The same diagnostic criteria apply to make the diagnosis of the clonal myeloproliferative disorders in children and adults (table 2) [29].

Table 2. WHO (2008) diagnostic criteria for Philadelphia chromosome-negative *BCR-ABL-1*-negative MPD

Myeloproliferative disorder	Diagnostic criteria
Essential Thrombocytosis[1] (ET)	(1) Sustained platelet count ≥450 × 10^9/l (2) Bone marrow biopsy showing excess enlarged, mature megakaryocytes; no significant increase or left shift of neutrophil granulopoiesis or erythropoiesis (3) Not meeting WHO criteria for polycythaemia vera, primary myelofibrosis, *BCR-ABL1*-positive chronic myelogenous leukaemia, myelodysplastic syndrome (4) Demonstration of *JAK2*V617F or other clonal marker; in the absence of *JAK2*V617F, no evidence for reactive thrombocytosis
Polycythaemia vera[2]	Major criteria (1) Haemoglobin >185 g/l in men or 165 g/l in women or other evidence of increased RBC volume (2) Presence of *JAK2*V617F or other functionally similar mutation such as *JAK2* exon 12 mutation Minor criteria (1) Bone marrow biopsy showing hypercellularity for age with trilineage growth (panmyelosis) with prominent erythroid, granulocytic, and megakaryocytic proliferation (2) Serum erythropoietin level below the reference range for normal; endogenous erythroid colony formation in vitro
Primary myelofibrosis[3]	Major criteria (1) Presence of megakaryocyte proliferation and atypia, accompanied by either reticulin and/or collagen fibrosis; in absence of significant reticulin fibrosis, a prefibrotic cellular-phase disease (2) Not meeting WHO criteria for polycythaemia vera, *BCR-ABL1*-positive chronic myelogenous leukaemia, myelodysplastic syndrome (3) Demonstration of *JAK2*V617F or other clonal marker (e.g. *MPL*W515K/L); in absence of clonal marker, no evidence of secondary bone marrow fibrosis Minor criteria (1) Leukoerythroblastosis (2) Increase in serum lactate dehydrogenase (3) Anaemia (4) Splenomegaly

[1] Diagnosis requires meeting all four criteria.
[2] Diagnosis requires the presence of both major criteria and one minor criterion or the presence of the first major criterion together with two minor criteria.
[3] Diagnosis requires meeting all three major and two minor criteria.

Genetics and Hereditary Predisposition

As with all myeloid neoplasms, next-generation sequencing technology is identifying key driver genes required to develop these neoplasms, which can occur either somatically or in the germline (de novo or inherited). In all children with suspected Philadelphia chromosome-negative *BCR-ABL1* MPD, a careful family history and search for mutations in genes implicated in these MPDs should be made in the child and family members.

In isolated cases and in pedigrees with elevated non-reactive platelet counts, activating germline mutations have been found in the genes encoding: (1) the stem cell/megakaryocyte lineage cytokine thrombopoietin (see [30] for additional references), (2) the thrombopoietin receptor *MPL* [31], and (3) one of the intracellular kinases downstream of the thrombopoietin receptor JAK2 (JAKV617I) [32]. There are numerous genetic causes of familial polycythaemia including mutations in: (1) the globin genes leading to high-affinity or methaemoglobin variants, (2) the erythropoietin receptor gene, and (3) the genes involved in oxygen sensing (e.g. *VHL* gene, *HIF2α* gene and the *PHD2* gene) (reviewed in [33]).

In addition to these germline mutations, a search should be made for the somatically mutated genes seen in ET, PV and PMF. These include *JAK2V617F*, *JAK2* exon 12 mutations, *MPLW515L* and rarely the epigenetic regulator *ASXL1* [7, 12].

In addition to the causal mutations described above, there is also a 5- to 7-fold risk of ET and PV in first-degree relatives of patients compared to controls and this has been attributed to a germline haplotype that includes the 3′ portion of the *JAK2* gene itself [34].

Finally, atypical chronic myeloid leukaemia and a related condition chronic neutrophilic leukaemia rarely seen in paediatric practice but more common in adults (so should be thought of in older adolescents) can have diagnostic activating mutations in the *CSF3R* gene (encoding the G-CSF receptor). Such patients could potentially respond to the JAK1/2 inhibitor ruxolitinib [35].

Presentation

Most children with polycythaemia present with a haemoglobin >180 g/l and non-specific symptoms. Though, rarely, children can present with thromboembolic disease particularly Budd-Chiari syndrome [7]. When children present with Budd-Chiari, they can often have normal haemoglobin though with an elevated red cell count but microcytic indices from iron deficiency. Children with primary myelofibrosis (PMF) present with cytopenia and require supportive therapy. Occasionally, patients with PMF can see spontaneous resolution of the condition. Importantly, there have been no described cases of acute leukaemic transformation in paediatric patients with ET, PV or PMF.

Therapy

For children with high platelet counts (this is the most common haematological finding in children) the risk of thromboembolism and haemorrhage is low. Cytoreductive therapy is rarely indicated unless there is a history of thromboembolism or haemorrhage. Interferon-α and hydroxycarbamide can both have significant side effects. Interferon-α can cause a flu-like syndrome, neuropsychiatric symptoms and autoimmune disorders. With hydroxycarbamide use, there is a potential concern of leukaemia from long-term use. Use of anti-platelet agents is also problematic. In children under 16 years of age, the use of aspirin should be considered with caution because of the risk of Reye's syndrome. In rare cases, especially PMF, haematopoietic stem cell transplantation has been an effective therapy in children with significant clinical problems due to cytopenia.

Primary Myelodysplasia Syndromes

Refractory Cytopenia of Childhood

Unlike DS-associated MPD/ML-DS and JMML, which are relatively well-defined disorders, the rest of paediatric myelodysplasia is very heterogeneous. Within sporadic MDS, RCC (reviewed in [36]) is most common, accounting for half the cases. Children with RCC present with symptoms secondary to anaemia, leucopenia and thrombocytopenia. Data from the European Working Group of MDS of Childhood shows that 75% of children have a platelet count $<150 \times 10^9$/l; 50% a neutrophil count of $<1 \times 10^9$/l and a haemoglobin of <100 g/l [37]. The marrow blast count is not increased. When there is a karyotypic abnormality the most common finding is monosomy 7 (10–20%) and this is associated with higher risk of progression to AML and an inferior survival [37]. However, in the majority of children with RCC the karyotype is normal. In addition, the marrow is usually hypocellular, unlike adult MDS.

Thus, separating RCC from cytopenia and hypocellularity due to other causes – for example, developing aplastic anaemia, infectious disease, immune-mediated cytopenia, metabolic disorders and inherited bone marrow failure disorders (see below) can be difficult. A trephine is often very helpful to accurately determine cellularity and help differentiate hypoplastic MDS from aplastic anaemia. As an example, in aplastic anaemia all three myeloid lineages are markedly reduced (erythroid, megakaryocytic and granulocytic), whereas in RCC there are usually clusters of erythroid islands (albeit with impaired maturation) with more profound reduction of megakaryocytic and granulocytic lineages.

For RCC there is no clear agreement of an optimal treatment strategy; the only curative therapy is stem cell transplantation. Timing of transplantation requires clinical judgment and careful discussion with the family. Acquisition of cytogenetic changes may predict transformation is an alert to proceed to transplantation but it important to remember that even children with a normal karyotype can progress to RAEB/RAEB-T and AML.

Refractory Anaemia with Excess Blasts and Refractory Anaemia with Excess Blasts in Transformation

A potential diagnostic challenge is to separate RAEB/RAEB-T from de novo AML. Though AML is defined as a blast count of >30%, biological features rather than a blast count cut-off are more important to clinical outcome and should guide decisions on therapeutic management. For example, children with a marrow blast count of <30% with recurrent cytogenetic abnormalities typically associated with de novo AML (e.g. t(8;21)(q22:q22) (*RUNX1-CBFA2T1*), inv(16) (p13q22) (*CBFB-MYH11*), t(15;17) (q22:q12) (*PML-RARα*) and t(9;11) (*MLL-MLLT3*)) should be treated as de novo AML, and not RAEB or RAEB-T, regardless of the blast count. In contrast, monosomy 7 is strongly suggestive of a diagnosis of MDS (see below) and should be treated as such. Finally, if there is any doubt and cytogenetic analyses do not provide a clue, it may be prudent to repeat the bone marrow after an interval of 2–4 weeks, depending on the peripheral blood count and film findings.

Prognostic scoring systems for childhood MDS are less developed compared with adults. In adults a number of scoring systems have been described and they include: (1) International Prognostic Scoring System (IPSS), (2) WHO classification-based prognostic scoring system, and (3) IPSS-revised. None of these systems is validated for children. In children, indicators of prognosis are the bone marrow blast count, cytogenetics, whether MDS is primary or secondary and a careful clinical assessment of the tempo of the disease. An abnormal karyotype is seen in ~55% of patients [38] and provides prognostic information in addition to confirming the diagnosis of abnormal clonal disorder. Monosomy 7 and/or 7q– are present in ~25% of the cases. Acquired trisomy 8 and 21 are the next most frequent. Children with a structurally complex karyotype with ≥3 numerical abnormalities including at least 1 structural change have a very poor outcome [38]. The outcome for patients with monosomy 7/7q is heterogeneous and influenced by the presence and nature of additional cytogenetic abnormalities [38].

RAEB and RAEB-T are challenging diseases to treat, like their adult counterparts. The only curative therapeutic approach is stem cell transplantation with some groups using course(s) of cytoreductive combination chemotherapy to prior to transplant [28, 39].

Secondary Myelodysplasia Syndromes

MDS can arise in children who have had chemotherapy and/or radiotherapy [28]. Secondary MDS is more common in children treated for epithelial tumours, more likely to occur in adolescents and typically occurs with a latency of 4–6 years from therapy. Secondary MDS is most commonly associated with monosomy 7 or *MLL* gene rearrangement. The outlook for patients with secondary MDS is poor, even with stem cell transplantation, with only 20–40% of children surviving ([40] and see references therein).

MDS can also occur on a background of an antecedent haematopoietic disorder such as aplastic anaemia, Fanconi anaemia, dyskeratosis congenita, Schwachman Diamond Bodian syndrome (SDBS), severe congential neutropenia and congential amegakaryocytic thromobocytopenia. Here an accurate appreciation of the relationship of the antecedent haematological disorder and MDS relies entirely on a careful history, examination, morphological assessment of the blood film, marrow, a requirement of >10% dysplasia in a cell lineage or in multiple lineages and specialist tests (e.g. Fanconi anaemia: chromosomal breakage tests and mutational analyses; dyskeratosis: genetic analysis of the telomerase RNA component TERC, the reverse transcriptase component TERT and the shelterin component TIN2; *SDBS* gene and the *TPO* gene for congential amegakaryocytic thromobocytopenia). A detailed discussion of aplastic anaemia and bone marrow failure disorders is beyond the scope of this article.

Familial MDS

There are rare pedigrees with cytopenias and morphological dysplasia. Within these pedigrees, mutations have been described within 6 genes that encode key regulators of haemopoiesis: *RUNX1* [41], *CEBPA* [42], *TERC* and *TERT* [43], *GATA2* ([44] and see therein for further references) and *GATA1* [45].

The ramifications of these studies are multiple. First, they show the power of molecular analysis to identify driver mutations in familial MDS, just as they have done in sporadic adult MDS (see above). This has allowed clinicians to begin to define clinical cytopenia and dysplastic conditions into molecular groups so as to define the clinical spectrum of a molecularly defined disease. This is analogous to the situation in JMML over the last decade. Second, they allow clinicians to identify germline variants and provide genetic counselling. Third, this detailed molecular characterisation is now being applied to sporadic paediatric myelodysplasia (both primary and secondary). Next generation sequencing – whole genome and exome – used in conjunction with conventional karyotyping and copy number analysis (e.g. by single nucleotide polymorphism arrays) will allow accurate genetic definition of disease – again a necessary prelude to defining more homogeneous clinical groups within paediatric MDS with better understanding of clinical course and prognosis.

References

1 Hasle H, Niemeyer CM, Chessells JM, et al: A pediatric approach to the WHO classification of myelodysplastic and myeloproliferative diseases. Leukemia 2003;17:277–282.

2 Baumann I, Niemeyer C, Bennett JM, Shannon K: Childhood myelodysplastic syndrome; in Swerdlow S, Campo E, Harris NL, et al (eds): WHO Classification of Tumours Of Haematopoietic and Lymphoid Tissues. Lyon, IARC, 2008, pp 104–107.

3 Hasle H, Niemeyer CM: Advances in the prognostication and management of advanced MDS in children. Br J Haematol 2011;154:185–195.
4 El-Moneim AA, Kratz CP, Boll S, Rister M, Pahl HL, Niemeyer CM: Essential versus reactive thrombocythemia in children: retrospective analyses of 12 cases. Pediatr Blood Cancer 2007;49:52–55.
5 Thiele J, Kvasnicka HM, Orazi A, Tefferi A, Gisslinger H: Essential thrombocythaemia; in Swerdlow H, Campo E, Harris NL, et al (eds): WHO Classification of Tumours of Haematopoietic and Lymphoid Tissues. Lyon, IARC, 2008, pp 48–50.
6 Thiele J, Kvasnicka HM, Orazi A, Tefferi A, Birgegard G: Polycthaemia vera; in Swerdlow H, Campo E, Harris NL, et al (eds): WHO Classification of Tumours of Haematopoietic and Lymphoid Tissues. Lyon, IARC, 2008, pp 40–43.
7 Cario H, Schwarz K, Herter JM, et al: Clinical and molecular characterisation of a prospectively collected cohort of children and adolescents with polycythemia vera. Br J Haematol 2008;142:622–626.
8 Thiele J, Kvasnicka HM, Tefferei A, Barosi G, Orazi A, Vardiman JW: Primary myelofibrosis; in Swerdlow SH, Campo E, Harris NL, et al (eds): Classification of Tumours of Haematopoietic and Lymphoid Tissues. Lyon, IARC, 2008, pp 44–47.
9 Campbell PJ, Green AR: The myeloproliferative disorders. N Engl J Med 2006;355:2452–2466.
10 Reilly JT, McMullin MF, Beer PA, et al: Guideline for the diagnosis and management of myelofibrosis. Br J Haematol 2012;158:453–471.
11 DeLario MR, Sheehan AM, Ataya R, et al: Clinical, histopathologic, and genetic features of pediatric primary myelofibrosis – an entity different from adults. Am J Hematol 2012;87:461–464.
12 Ismael O, Shimada A, Hama A, et al: Mutations profile of polycythemia vera and essential thrombocythemia among Japanese children. Pediatr Blood Cancer 2012;59:530–535.
13 Roy A, Roberts I, Vyas P: Biology and management of transient abnormal myelopoiesis (TAM) in children with Down syndrome. Semin Fetal Neonatal Med 2012;17:196–201.
14 Massey GV, Zipursky A, Chang MN, et al: A prospective study of the natural history of transient leukemia (TL) in neonates with Down syndrome (DS): Children's Oncology Group (COG) study POG-9481. Blood 2006;107:4606–4613.
15 Klusmann JH, Creutzig U, Zimmermann M, et al: Treatment and prognostic impact of transient leukemia in neonates with Down syndrome. Blood 2008; 111:2991–2998.
16 Gamis AS, Alonzo TA, Gerbing RB, et al: Natural history of transient myeloproliferative disorder clinically diagnosed in Down syndrome neonates: a report from the Children's Oncology Group Study A2971. Blood 2011;118:6752–6759; quiz 6996.
17 Hasle H, Abrahamsson J, Arola M, et al: Myeloid leukemia in children 4 years or older with Down syndrome often lacks GATA1 mutation and cytogenetics and risk of relapse are more akin to sporadic AML. Leukemia 2007;22:1428–1430.
18 Ahmed M, Sternberg A, Hall G, et al: Natural history of GATA1 mutations in Down syndrome. Blood 2004;103:2480–2489.
19 Roy A, Roberts I, Norton A, Vyas P: Acute megakaryoblastic leukaemia (AMKL) and transient myeloproliferative disorder (TMD) in Down syndrome: a multi-step model of myeloid leukaemogenesis. Br J Haematol 2009;147:3–12.
20 Sorrell AD, Alonzo TA, Hilden JM, et al: Favorable survival maintained in children who have myeloid leukemia associated with Down syndrome using reduced-dose chemotherapy on Children's Oncology Group trial A2971:a report from the Children's Oncology Group. Cancer 2012;118:4806–4814.
21 Pine SR, Guo Q, Yin C, Jayabose S, Druschel CM, Sandoval C: Incidence and clinical implications of GATA1 mutations in newborns with Down syndrome. Blood 2007;110:2128–2131.
22 Bull MJ: Health supervision for children with Down syndrome. Pediatrics 2011;128:393–406.
23 Roy A, Cowan G, Mead AJ, et al: Perturbation of fetal liver hematopoietic stem and progenitor cell development by trisomy 21. Proc Natl Acad Sci USA 2012; 109:17579–17584.
24 Sankaran VG, Ghazvinian R, Do R, et al: Exome sequencing identifies GATA1 mutations resulting in Diamond-Blackfan anemia. J Clin Invest 2012;122: 2439–2443.
25 Loh ML: Recent advances in the pathogenesis and treatment of juvenile myelomonocytic leukaemia. Br J Haematol 2011;152:677–687.
26 Romano AA, Allanson JE, Dahlgren J, et al: Noonan syndrome: clinical features, diagnosis, and management guidelines. Pediatrics 2010;126:746–759.
27 Niemeyer CM, Kang MW, Shin DH, et al: Germline CBL mutations cause developmental abnormalities and predispose to juvenile myelomonocytic leukemia. Nat Genet 2010;42:794–800.
28 Kobos R, Steinherz PG, Kernan NA, et al: Allogeneic hematopoietic stem cell transplantation for pediatric patients with treatment-related myelodysplastic syndrome or acute myelogenous leukemia. Biol Blood Marrow Transplant 2012;18:473–480.
29 Barbui T, Barosi G, Birgegard G, et al: Philadelphia-negative classical myeloproliferative neoplasms: critical concepts and management recommendations from European LeukemiaNet. J Clin Oncol 2011;29: 761–770.
30 Liu K, Kralovics R, Rudzki Z, et al: A de novo splice donor mutation in the thrombopoietin gene causes hereditary thrombocythemia in a Polish family. Haematologica 2008;93:706–714.

31 Liu K, Martini M, Rocca B, et al: Evidence for a founder effect of the MPL-S505N mutation in eight Italian pedigrees with hereditary thrombocythemia. Haematologica 2009;94:1368–1374.
32 Mead AJ, Chowdhury O, Pecquet C, et al: Impact of isolated germline JAK2V617I mutation on human hematopoiesis. Blood 2013;121:4156–4165.
33 Patnaik MM, Tefferi A: The complete evaluation of erythrocytosis: congenital and acquired. Leukemia 2009;23:834–844.
34 Jones AV, Campbell PJ, Beer PA, et al: The JAK2 46/1 haplotype predisposes to MPL-mutated myeloproliferative neoplasms. Blood 2010;115:4517–4523.
35 Pardanani A, Lasho TL, Laborde RR, et al: CSF3R T618I is a highly prevalent and specific mutation in chronic neutrophilic leukemia. Leukemia 2013, epub ahead of print.
36 Niemeyer CM, Baumann I: Classification of childhood aplastic anemia and myelodysplastic syndrome. Hematology 2011;2011:84–89.
37 Kardos G, Baumann I, Passmore SJ, et al: Refractory anemia in childhood: a retrospective analysis of 67 patients with particular reference to monosomy 7. Blood 2003;102:1997–2003.
38 Gohring G, Michalova K, Beverloo HB, et al: Complex karyotype newly defined: the strongest prognostic factor in advanced childhood myelodysplastic syndrome. Blood 2010;116:3766–3769.
39 Kikuchi A, Hasegawa D, Ohtsuka Y, et al: Outcome of children with refractory anaemia with excess of blast (RAEB) and RAEB in transformation (RAEB-T) in the Japanese MDS99 study. Br J Haematol 2012; 158:657–661.
40 Aguilera DG, Vaklavas C, Tsimberidou AM, Wen S, Medeiros LJ, Corey SJ: Pediatric therapy-related myelodysplastic syndrome/acute myeloid leukemia: the MD Anderson Cancer Center experience. J Pediatr Hematol Oncol 2009;31:803–811.
41 Song WJ, Sullivan MG, Legare RD, et al: Haploinsufficiency of CBFA2 causes familial thrombocytopenia with propensity to develop acute myelogenous leukaemia. Nat Genet 1999;23:166–175.
42 Pabst T, Eyholzer M, Haefliger S, Schardt J, Mueller BU: Somatic CEBPA mutations are a frequent second event in families with germline CEBPA mutations and familial acute myeloid leukemia. J Clin Oncol 2008;26:5088–5093.
43 Kirwan M, Vulliamy T, Marrone A, et al: Defining the pathogenic role of telomerase mutations in myelodysplastic syndrome and acute myeloid leukemia. Hum Mutat 2009;30:1567–1573.
44 Bodor C, Renneville A, Smith M, et al: Germ-line GATA2 p.THR354MET mutation in familial myelodysplastic syndrome with acquired monosomy 7 and ASXL1 mutation demonstrating rapid onset and poor survival. Haematologica 2012;97:890–894.
45 Hollanda LM, Lima CS, Cunha AF, et al: An inherited mutation leading to production of only the short isoform of GATA-1 is associated with impaired erythropoiesis. Nat Genet 2006;38:807–812.

Prof. Paresh Vyas
Department of Haematology and MRC Molecular Haematology Unit
Weatherall Institute of Molecular Medicine
Oxford OX3 9DS (UK)
E-Mail paresh.vyas@imm.ox.ac.uk

Thomas AE, Halsey C (eds): Controversies in Pediatric and Adolescent Hematology.
Pediatr Adolesc Med. Basel, Karger, 2014, vol 17, pp 98–115 (DOI: 10.1159/000350349)

Towards Personalised Medicine in Childhood Acute Lymphoblastic Leukaemia

Christina Halsey

Institute of Infection, Immunity and Inflammation, College of Medical, Veterinary and Life Sciences, Glasgow Biomedical Research Centre, University of Glasgow, Glasgow, UK

Abstract

Childhood leukaemia is one of the success stories of modern medicine. Initially advances were made by using progressively more intensive multi-agent chemotherapy regimens for all children. More recently, it has been appreciated that individual children differ considerably with respect to the sensitivity of their leukaemic cells to chemotherapy and also their susceptibility to treatment-related toxicity. This has led to a move towards more personalised treatment. The mainstay of this approach is the use of minimal residual disease measurement which assesses each patient's response to initial therapy and enables treatment modifications to be made in real time. Personalised approaches also extend to identifying children at risk of drug toxicity using pharmacogenomics and the use of molecular techniques to identify mutations in leukaemic cells that can be specifically targeted by new drugs. This article reviews the techniques and strategies in current use and speculates on how advances in interpreting the explosion of genetic information becoming available may improve treatment for children with leukaemia in the future. Copyright © 2014 S. Karger AG, Basel

The treatment of childhood acute lymphoblastic leukaemia (ALL) is a modern-day success story. From an almost universally fatal disease in the 1950s and 1960s, a child diagnosed with ALL today can expect a cure rate greater than 85% [1, 2]. The chemotherapy drugs used to tackle ALL have remained essentially unchanged for the last 30 years so what underlies this remarkable achievement? Study of progressive therapeutic trials has shown that step-wise improvement between 1960 and the 1990s has occurred largely due to better scheduling of drugs, recognition of the need to provide adequate therapy directed against disease in the central nervous system and the advent of much improved supportive care. The latter includes not only the availability of new antimicrobial and antifungal medications and formulations but also advances in our understanding of how and when to deliver these drugs, with a shift from use in confirmed infections to pre-emptive and prophylactic use.

Another reason for improved outcomes is the willingness by physicians and families to accept more toxicity from drug treatment in anticipation of a greater chance of cure. Treatment for leukaemia remains highly intensive with a small but significant risk of treatment related mortality particularly due to infective deaths. We are now at the point where the risk of death from the treatment is nearly equivalent to the risk of death from relapsed leukaemia – particularly in patients with so-called 'low-risk' disease. This has necessitated a paradigm shift in leukaemia treatment protocols. Previous trials generally compared the current gold-standard drug combination with a combination of drugs (usually more intensive) that might improve leukaemic cell kill. However, since the early 2000s leukaemia trials have started to address whether treatment intensity can actually be reduced for some groups of children. In this article, the ways in which this has been achieved will be reviewed as well as discussion as to how further advances might be made in 'individualising' treatment for leukaemia. Of course it should not be forgotten that despite this remarkable success story there are also children whose disease is extremely difficult to treat. New advances that might help these patients will be discussed.

Overview of Acute Lymphoblastic Leukaemia Therapy

In 1948, it was first reported that temporary remissions could be induced in ALL using anti-folate drugs [3]. Further active agents were soon identified, but the next real advance came when it was discovered that the use of multiple chemotherapy agents given over a prolonged period in different combinations, so-called 'total therapy', rather than use of single agents could produce long-term remissions and even cure in some patients [4]. Thus, ALL became the first human cancer to be cured by drug therapy alone. The total therapy regimens used in the 1950s still remain the backbone of modern day leukaemia protocols consisting of an induction phase to produce disease remission followed by consolidation and intensification blocks, central nervous system (CNS) directed therapy and continuing therapy to maintain remission.

The mainstay of drug therapy for ALL comprises corticosteroids (prednisolone or dexamethasone), vinca alkaloids (chiefly vincristine), asparaginase, antifolates (methotrexate), anthracyclines (such as daunorubicin) and purine analogues (6-mercaptopurine). Although chemotherapy protocols vary in their exact details between different international trial groups they are broadly comparable. The main phases of treatment are briefly described below.

Remission Induction

Induction therapy aims to eradicate more than 99% of the leukaemic cell burden and restore normal haematopoiesis by the end of 4–6 weeks of therapy. It consists of a combination of corticosteroids, vincristine and asparaginase. These drugs form the cornerstone of induction because they are non-myelosuppressive, synergistic and target different anticancer pathways. Anthracyclines can be added but these are potentially toxic and myelosuppressive and therefore associated with greater morbidity; for this reason they are often reserved for patients with higher risk disease.

Consolidation and Intensification

The next phase of therapy aims to consolidate and/or intensify the treatment to eradicate the remaining 1% or so of leukaemic cells. These cells have survived the original induction therapy and therefore combinations of different anti-leukaemia drugs are used at this stage to try and circumvent drug resistance. There is currently no consensus on the best regimens or their duration but it is generally accepted that 'stronger not longer' therapy is best – especially for higher risk disease. This phase of therapy consists of consolidation and delayed intensification blocks and some form of CNS directed therapy. Methotrexate, cyclophosphamide, cytarabine and asparaginase usually play key roles.

Central Nervous System Prophylaxis

Soon after the introduction of systemic therapy for ALL it became clear that despite effective bone marrow clearance of disease, up to 75% of children would rapidly relapse with leukaemic blasts in the CNS. To prevent this, treatment was introduced to eliminate leukaemic cells at this site. Initially, this consisted of cranial or craniospinal irradiation, but concerns were raised over the toxic effects of this treatment as discussed below. There has now been a shift to the use of intrathecal chemotherapy and systemic drugs with good CNS penetration in place of radiotherapy without compromising efficacy [1].

Maintenance Therapy

The prolonged administration of relatively low dose chemotherapy during a maintenance phase lasting 1–3 years is almost unique to ALL. However, attempts to omit this phase or shorten it below 12 months have led to significantly greater rates of relapse. The reasons why maintenance is required for long-term cure are currently unknown although it may hint at a population of long lived, slow cycling leukaemia-initiating cells. Combinations of oral 6-mercaptopurine (6MP) and methotrexate with or without pulses of vincristine and corticosteroids make up the backbone of this treatment phase.

Burden of Treatment

The treatment strategies described above underlie the remarkable improvement in ALL survival rates, but at what cost? The potential for significant long-term sequelae from ALL treatment was first recognised very early on when it became clear that use of cranial irradiation in young children (particularly those under 2 years of age) could result in significant toxicity. CNS-directed treatment can produce neurocognitive impairment although the precise contributions of systemic chemotherapy, intrathecal treatment and radiotherapy are unclear and most children treated on modern protocols have IQ scores within the normal range [5]. Cranial irradiation is also known to produce a high rate of second malignancies in the CNS as well as significant endocrinopathies. Taken together this has led to removal of cranial irradiation from many current treatment protocols [1].

Major toxicities still occur, both acutely during treatment and as 'late effects'. The global effects of intensive treatment produce profound immunosuppression leading to an increased risk of death related to fungal and bacterial pathogens (particularly Gram-negative sepsis). In addition, individual therapeutic agents, either alone or in combination, have specific side effects such as avascular necrosis (mainly steroid related), acute pancreatitis (steroids and asparaginase), cerebral venous sinus thrombosis (asparaginase), encephalopathy (methotrexate and cytarabine) and peripheral neuropathy (vinca alkaloids). These toxicities are commoner and more severe in children on more intensive regimens but are also highly age dependent with adolescents suffering many more significant grade 3 and 4 toxicities than younger children.

Taken together, the burden of these individual toxicities is high, particularly in older patients. Toxicity has generally increased over time since advances in supportive care have allowed more intensive scheduling of drugs and uses of higher doses or more potent formulations. Recent ALL trials suggest that in good-risk patients, the risk of treatment-related mortality is approaching the risk of death due to relapsed disease [2]. However, we know that in historical trials with much less intensive protocols, such as the UKALL VII trial which finished in 1980 and only had one block of delayed intensification, approximately 50% of patients were cured. Over the last 30 years progressive intensification of treatment has benefited the remaining 35–40% of patients but at the expense of theoretically overtreating the 50% of patients who would have been cured with less-intensive protocols. These observations have led to a move towards tailored treatment for patients, i.e. reductions in treatment for patients with 'good-risk' disease, with the aim of limiting exposure to drugs with the potential for prolonged immunosuppression, major organ toxicity or promotion of secondary malignancy. Conversely identification of patients with poor risk disease may allow further treatment intensification and/or adoption of novel treatment strategies.

Risk Stratification in Childhood ALL

The aim of tailored therapy is to be able to identify prospectively how sensitive the disease (and the patient) will be to treatment and use this information to adjust therapy accordingly. Risk stratification into poor- and standard-risk disease has been used for many years based on clinical variables such as age and presenting white cell count. More recently, cytogenetic abnormalities have been identified that add to this assessment. The major clinical and biological features in routine use to classify children at initial presentation are discussed below.

Clinical Factors

Age is a major prognostic variable; with children aged 1–9 having consistently better outcomes than infants (aged 0–1) and older children/adolescents. This partly reflects the distribution of different leukaemia cytogenetic subtypes in different age groups (and therefore relates to the leukaemia biologic features discussed below). However, even within a defined subgroup such as Philadelphia positive ALL (Ph+ve ALL) (where the chromosomal translocation t(9;22) is present in the lymphoblasts) children do better than adolescents, who in turn fare better than adults. Interestingly, adolescents treated on adult leukaemia protocols do consistently worse than those treated on paediatric protocols [6] implying that the chemotherapy regimen is an important determinant of outcome.

Presenting white cell count influences prognosis, especially for precursor-B (pre-B) cell disease with counts $>50 \times 10^9/l$ used as the cut off for a higher risk group. Very high white cell counts may produce direct toxicity such as leucostasis, but the reasons behind the adverse prognosis of even moderately elevated white cell counts as a continuous variable are not clear. In T cell disease counts $>100 \times 10^9/l$ are associated with CNS infiltration but lower counts have less prognostic significance.

Biological Features

ALL can be subclassified according to its cell of origin: pre-B, mature B or T cell. Although T cell disease has traditionally fared worse than B cell disease, this prognostic feature has largely been eliminated by modern intensive treatment protocols. In addition, cytogenetic analysis of leukaemic blasts allows identification of acquired genetic abnormalities. Major advances have been made in identifying and understanding the prognostic significance of the myriad chromosomal abnormalities, both numerical and structural found by such analysis [7]. Cytogenetic abnormalities such as the possession of >50 chromosomes per cell (high hyperdiploidy) or the t(12;21) translocation can be good risk, i.e. associated with an excellent outcome with conventional treatment. Others are considered poor risk such as near haploidy (23–29 chromosomes per cell) or presence of a t(4;11) *(AF4-MLL)* translocation. As seen with many other variables, the high-risk group only accounts for small numbers of patients, so although it is highly predictive of poor outcome in these patients, the majority of relapses occur in the numerically much larger good- and standard-risk groups.

With the sequencing of the human genome and the advent of high throughput technology, an increasing amount of molecular genetic information is becoming available; this is discussed in more detail below.

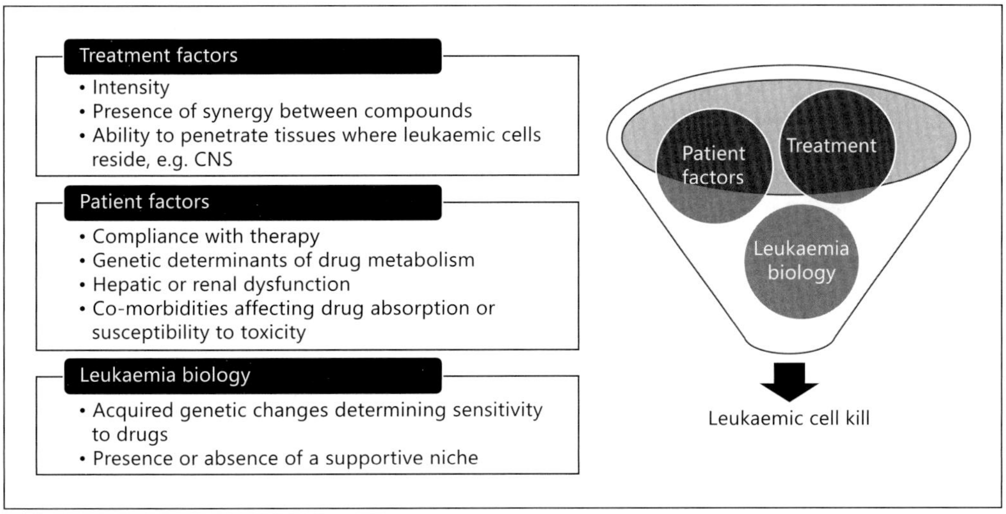

Fig. 1. Factors that determine leukaemic cell kill.

Identification of a 'Personalised' Risk

The clinical and biological risk factors described above are still in widespread use and form the US National Cancer Institute risk stratification used by many trial groups for initial choice of induction therapy (usually 3 vs. 4 drug inductions with addition of an anthracycline for higher risk patients). Although these criteria are reasonably predictive of high- and low-risk disease on a population scale, they are insufficiently sensitive to determine an individual child's risk of relapse. Indeed, the majority of children fall in the standard risk group and, although their relapse rate is proportionally much lower than high-risk children, they make up numerically the largest group of relapses. Therefore, it would make no sense to globally reduce therapy for standard risk children based on these criteria alone as the number of relapses would inevitably rise.

Another major limitation of standard epidemiological approaches is that the strongest predictor of relapse is the treatment given. With the increased intensity of modern treatment protocols many features that were previously considered high risk, such as male sex and T cell disease, have lost their prognostic significance. Therefore, approaches that take into account the chemotherapy delivered are essential.

Overall, the response to treatment involves interplay between the intrinsic biological properties of individual leukaemic clones, the child's pharmacogenomic make-up and additional factors such as the exact dose and scheduling of chemotherapeutic agents, compliance with therapy and/or presence of co-existing pathology. This is illustrated in figure 1. These complex and sometimes unmeasurable variables limit the use of risk scores and other algorithms to individualise treatment. Instead, focus has shifted to measuring the end result of all these variables, i.e. the degree of leukaemic cell kill after an initial phase of therapy in an individual child. This approach has been termed minimal residual disease (MRD) detection.

Measuring response to therapy in vivo is not a new concept – variables such as the reduction of peripheral blast count in response to a 7-day steroid pre-phase (widely used by the international Berlin-Frankfurt-Munster (iBFM) trial group), or the number of blasts in the bone marrow after 8, 15 or 28 days of therapy, have been used for many years. However, MRD represents a major advance because of the high sensitivity it affords. Bone marrow examination under the light microscope by an experienced haematologist can identify between 1 and 5 leukaemic cells per 100 bone marrow cells examined (i.e. 1–5% leukaemic blasts). However, leukaemic blasts can be difficult to distinguish from normal regenerating bone marrow precursors and this limits the specificity of this approach. In addition, the vast majority of children, including most of those destined to relapse later during treatment, will have reached this level of morphological remission at the end of induction therapy making this approach too insensitive to detect poor responders. Sensitivity has been greatly improved by using flow cytometry or PCR-based approaches to detect residual leukaemic cells. This is 100–10,000 times more sensitive than light microscopy. Therefore, whilst more than 95% of children have achieved morphological remission by the end of 28 days of induction therapy, approximately 50% of them will still have some detectable disease using more sensitive MRD-based techniques [8].

There are two main techniques used to measure MRD; flow cytometry identifies and tracks leukaemic cells based on aberrant expression of proteins on the cell surface, whilst PCR-based methods are used to track genetic alterations in leukaemic clones at the DNA or RNA level. These two methods have different pros and cons [9, 10]. In order to be a good marker of MRD, assays need to be sensitive (although the degree of sensitivity required depends on the time-point being tested), specific (to enable discrimination between leukaemic cells and normal BM counterparts to prevent false positive results), quantifiable, stable over time (to prevent false negative results), reproducible between labs to allow use in multi-centre trials, and also available promptly to allow treatment decisions to be made. The main methods in use are reviewed below.

Flow Cytometry

Leukaemic cells often express proteins on their cell surfaces that are not seen in normal lymphocytes at the same developmental stage. Staining leukaemic cells and normal bone marrow cells with a panel of antibodies directed against these aberrant proteins allows identification of combinations of antigens which are only co-expressed in leukaemic cells and not in normal bone marrow. This is termed a leukaemia-associated immunophenotype (LAIP). Once a LAIP has been defined it can be used to track leukaemic cells over time. This method tends to have high clinical applicability in that a LAIP can be identified in over 95% of children with ALL. Flow cytometry is relatively cheap and widely available and therefore this technique is attractive to clinicians in smaller units. However, choice of markers and interpretation of results requires significant expertise. For example, it is possible that the leukaemic cells will down-regulate cell-surface proteins when exposed to treatment and therefore no longer be recognised. Attempts to track disease in laboratories with insufficient expertise reduce both the specificity and sensitivity of this test. This can be improved by local processing and acquisition of data using standardised operating procedures followed by expert analysis at central laboratories [8, 9].

Flow cytometry is about 10-fold less sensitive than PCR with average detection rates of about 1 leukaemic cell per 10,000 normal BM cells. This is not necessarily a disadvantage if the technique is being used at early time-points.

PCR Based Methods

There are two main PCR-based methods in use (1) PCR-based tracking of immunoglobulin and T cell receptor gene rearrangements, and (2) use of PCR to track leukaemia-associated fusion transcripts.

Immunoglobulin and T Cell Receptor Gene Rearrangements. During early B and T cell development, immunoglobulin and T cell receptor genes undergo rearrangement in order to generate unique antigen recognition sites. This involves random combinatorial use of three different gene segments: the variable region (V), diversity region (D) and the junctional region (J). In addition, the process introduces basepair changes in the native DNA sequence to generate further diversity. The end result is that each lymphocyte possesses a unique coding sequence in the VDJ region which results in the vast array of antigen recognition sites needed to provide defence against invading micro-organisms. This unique VDJ sequence can act as a 'fingerprint' marking each lymphocyte and all its progeny. Identification of this fingerprint is the basis for PCR immunoglobulin/T cell receptor MRD measurement. In the laboratory patients, leukaemic blasts are isolated from diagnostic bone marrow specimens and the VDJ gene segments of the leukaemic cells are identified and sequenced. This information is used to design patient-specific PCR primers that will only bind to the unique fingerprint region. Leukaemic clones can then be tracked using quantitative PCR. At least two different markers are used to monitor disease progress to guard against continuing rearrangements in the genetic material of leukaemic cells during treatment (clonal evolution), or the existence of multiple clones. As can be appreciated, this technique is quite laborious and requires significant expertise, making it relatively expensive and unsuitable for smaller laboratories. In addition, it is impossible to identify reliable and sensitive markers in all patients although it has clinical applicability in more than 90% of patients [10]. This technique is much more sensitive than flow cytometry with the ability to detect 1 leukaemic cell per 10,000–100,000 normal bone marrow cells. In addition it is very accurate and provides robust quantitative information over time.

Leukaemia-Associated Fusion Transcripts. Some leukaemias carry recurring fusion transcripts such as the t(9;22) *BCR-ABL* translocation or t(12;21) *TEL-AML1*. Probes and primers can be designed to detect the fusion transcript and the level of this transcript can be followed over time. This technique is limited by the fact that only about

40% of patients have a suitable fusion transcript. In these patients, it is a sensitive rapid technique and has the advantage of measuring a variable that has a direct and unequivocal link with the leukaemic clone. However, RNA is less stable than DNA so this technique is more affected by poor sample quality which may produce false-negative results. This technique is in routine use for patients with the *BCR-ABL* translocation (discussed in more detail below), but is not widely used for other ALL fusion proteins at present.

Importance of Treatment Protocol and Time-Point

It is worth noting that since MRD measures the response to a given treatment in an individual patient it is therefore, by definition, extremely treatment dependent. For example the levels of MRD measured after 15 days of treatment are likely to be much lower, even in the same patient with the same leukaemic clone, if the patient has received 4 drugs rather than 3 in this period. This means that the exact level of MRD that predicts good- or poor-risk disease (such as less than 0.001% leukaemic cells after 1 month of treatment) cannot be directly extrapolated to different treatment protocols. Similarly, the level of MRD that represents a good or poor response to treatment will depend on the time-point at which the MRD is measured, e.g. levels such as 1 leukaemic cell per 100 normal cells might be considered good risk after 15 days of treatment but would be ultra-high risk after 11 weeks of treatment.

Clinical Studies Measuring MRD

Numerous studies involving thousands of patients have established that MRD can reliably identify good and poor risk patients amongst children with ALL [8, 10, 11]. The level of MRD after initial therapy is the strongest prognostic variable in virtually all studies and renders almost all traditional prognostic markers redundant [8]. The value of MRD was first proven for pre-B ALL but has also been found to predict outcome for T-ALL, Ph+ve ALL and other cytogenetic subtypes that have been examined in sufficient numbers [10]. It also appears to have prognostic significance in relapsed disease with MRD levels predicting response to both chemotherapy and haematopoietic stem cell transplant (HSCT). However, to really revolutionise the outcome for patients, it is important to be able to show that measurement of MRD has led to superior outcomes. Recent leukaemia trials have been addressing this; particularly whether the presence of low risk MRD can be used to safely de-escalate treatment and/or whether the outcome for high risk disease can be improved by its prospective identification and subsequent treatment intensification. For example, in the UKALL2003 study, children were stratified according to day 28 MRD results. Low-risk children (MRD negative at day 28) were eligible for a randomisation between the standard two blocks of intensification therapy or a treatment reduction to one block. High-risk children (MRD $>10^{-4}$ at day 28) were randomised to staying on their current treatment arm or moving up to the most intensive arm in an attempt to prevent relapse. Treatment reduction for low risk children was safe and effective and therefore this randomisation was stopped early and all subsequent patients with low risk MRD were allocated one block of intensification [11]. The high-risk randomisation has not yet achieved sufficient patient accrual or follow-up to give definitive results. However, data from elsewhere are accumulating to support increased treatment intensity in patients with high risk MRD [1, 12].

Can MRD Be Used as an Outcome Measure?
The success of modern ALL therapy has resulted in very low relapse rates. Whilst this is obviously a cause for celebration, on a practical level it makes it increasingly difficult to evaluate new treatments using traditional endpoints such as relapse rate and 5- and 10-year survival data. The low rate of events means that very large numbers of participants are required to prove superiority of one treatment versus another. This difficulty is compounded by the fact that many new drugs are targeted at small subgroups of high risk patients so the pool of eligible patients is very small. In an attempt to speed up the development and testing of new drug compounds for leukaemia the issue has arisen as to whether MRD measurement can be used as a surrogate marker for treatment efficacy. Although tempting, this has not yet been validated and a number of observations suggest it should be treated with caution. Firstly, several independent trials have noted that, despite its excellent overall prognostic utility, bone marrow levels of MRD are a poor predictor of extramedullary relapse, with non-marrow (e.g. isolated CNS) relapses occurring in low-risk and high-risk MRD patients with almost equal frequency in some reports [12]. Secondly, the recently reported UK ALLR3 trial for relapsed and refractory ALL showed a significantly better Event Free Survival (EFS) for induction therapy using mitoxantrone versus idarubicin despite no differences in day 28 MRD levels between the two randomised arms [13].

Further Personalised Approaches

Personalised therapy does not stop at the use of MRD for risk stratification. Other approaches currently in use include:

1 Identification of an individual's susceptibility to drug effects and toxicity.
2 Identification of individual therapeutic targets.
3 Identification of additional prognostic factors using molecular genetics.

These will be discussed in the following sections.

Personalised Pharmacology

As discussed above, children with ALL are vulnerable to a multitude of drug-related toxicities which may be dose related or due to inherited or acquired susceptibility. A major goal of personalised medicine is to tailor therapy to minimise side effects whilst maximising efficacy. This approach is clearly not new; paediatric drugs have always been dosed according to variables such as age, weight, and more recently adjustments for BMI have been introduced. Unfortunately, the majority of cancer drugs have a low therapeutic index, i.e. a narrow (or overlapping) window between an effective therapeutic dose and a toxic dose. If all patients receive the same mg/kg drug dose then a dose has to be chosen that balances the risk of serious toxicity in sensitive patients with the risk of significantly underdosing other patients and thereby increasing their risk of relapse. This is where individualised dosing can play a major role, using patient specific information to set a dose that avoids toxicity whilst maximising therapeutic effect. Early trials provided proof of principle; children with pre-B ALL randomly assigned to individualised methotrexate dosing based on their measured drug clearance had better outcomes than children assigned to conventional dosing based on body surface area [14].

In order to fully implement personalised pharmacology, it is necessary to have knowledge of the major drug activating and inactivating pathways and be able to measure these in some way as well as an understanding of the genetic and environmental factors that determine both drug efficacy and end-organ susceptibility to toxicity. Although we are a long way from a complete knowledge of all these complex effects, major advances have been made over the last two decades. Sequencing of the human genome, advent of high throughput genetic testing and increased understanding of drug metabolism have opened the way for a huge array of available tests. Knowing how and when to use these tests remains a challenge but has the potential for enormous benefit. An example of this is analysis of the thiopurine methyltransferase *(TPMT)* genotype.

TPMT activity is by far the best-characterised genetic determinant of drug sensitivity in ALL. This enzyme catalyzes the intracellular inactivation of thiopurines (azathioprine, 6MP and 6-thioguanine). Family studies have identified that some individuals carry non-functional *TPMT* alleles and that enzyme activity is inherited as an autosomal co-dominant trait. Therefore, it is possible to possess 1 of 3 genotypes: (1) homozygous wild-type, with normal enzyme levels, seen in about 90% of the population, (2) heterozygous deficiency with TPMT levels varying between 30 and 60% of normal, seen in about 10% of the population, or (3) homozygous deficiency leading to undetectable enzyme levels, seen in about 1 in 300 patients (or at even lower frequency in some ethnic groups).

Clinical studies have linked severe (and even fatal) haematological toxicity to homozygous TPMT deficiency. It is now common to carry out *TPMT* genotyping at the onset of treatment and start with a reduced dosing schedule for patients with homozygous or heterozygous deficiency [15]. This has led to a reduced incidence of severe toxicity.

Of note, although individualised thiopurine dosing to reduce toxicity may be effective this cannot necessarily be extrapolated to other situations. For example, the NOPHO trial group tested whether measurement of thiopurine metabolites alongside measures of BM suppression could be used to escalate 6MP doses to improve EFS. Unfortunately this approach resulted in no improvement in boys and an increased relapse rate in girls, attributed to possible effects of methylated 6MP metabolites promoting leukaemic cell dormancy [16].

Personalised Therapeutic Targets

Although most leukaemia is treated according to a standard schedule, the ability to better characterise the genetic basis for leukaemia and identify antigens expressed on the surface of leukaemic cells has allowed some new therapies to be developed. Only patients carrying the corresponding target will benefit from such directed therapy and therefore this treatment is also individualised. Two examples are given below.

Philadelphia Positive ALL

The Philadelphia chromosome consists of a reciprocal translocation between the Abelson oncogene (*ABL*) on chromosome 9 and the breakpoint cluster region *(BCR)* on chromosome 22 to produce a fusion oncoprotein BCR-ABL. This oncoprotein has constitutive tyrosine kinase activity and is one of the key drivers for the development and maintenance of leukaemia. Two different breakpoints, p190 and p210, in the *BCR* gene are associated with ALL and chronic myeloid leukaemia, respectively. The discovery of imatinib, a tyrosine kinase inhibitor, has greatly improved the outlook for patients with Ph+ve ALL. Imatinib was initially developed as a treatment for chronic myeloid leukaemia but was later shown to have activity in Ph+ve ALL. About 3% of children with ALL have Ph+ve disease and this translocation confers poor risk. Although mature data are not yet available, early results suggest that addition of imatinib can significantly improve response rates. In a US Children's Oncology Group (COG) study, 50 children treated with imatinib plus chemotherapy and/or HSCT had a 3-year EFS of 80 ± 11%, more than twice historical controls (35 ± 4%; $p < 0.0001$), with no apparent toxicities seen on adding imatinib to already intensive chemotherapy regimens [17]. In addition, the 3-year EFS was similar for patients treated with chemotherapy plus imatinib (88 ± 11%; 95% CI 66–96%) or sibling donor BMT (57 ± 22%; 95% CI 30.4–76.1%), although it should be noted that this study excluded the highest risk patients, those with induction failure [17]. These encouraging early results have been followed up by a recent report from a European Intergroup randomised trial, EsPhALL [18]. In this trial, Ph+ve ALL patients aged 1–18 were allocated to good- and poor-risk groups according to early treatment responses which were defined using the standard criteria of peripheral blast count after 7 days of prednisolone therapy and blast counts on a day 8/15 BM and day 28 BM. Good-risk patients (rapid early responders) were randomised to post-induction chemotherapy with or without imatinib, whilst poor risk patients (slow early responders) all received imatinib plus conventional chemotherapy. In the randomised comparison, the imatinib group showed improved disease-free survival at 4 years (72.9 vs. 61.7%) although this only reached statistical significance when analyzed by actual treatment rather than intention to treat. In the poor-risk group, which included patients with induction failure, 4-year disease-free survival was 53.5%, compared with 29.7% in historical controls. Again, no significant additional toxicities were attributable to imatinib. This trial had to be stopped early due to publication of the COG study [17] and data emerging from adult studies making parents and children unwilling to accept the 'no imatinib' arm. This illustrates the problems of definitively testing new drugs for poor prognosis subsets of ALL; large collaborative studies are needed to achieve sufficient patient numbers, compliance to the study protocol is often poor and rapid end-points may be needed if trial objectives are to be met.

By monitoring the number of *BCR-ABL* transcripts using quantitative PCR, it is possible to define whether children have achieved a molecular as well as cytogenetic remission following treatment. There is now discussion as to whether transplantation can be safely omitted from children with good risk MRD and this is currently being tested in a European trial using the more potent tyrosine kinase inhibitor dasatinib rather than imatinib to target *BCR-ABL*. Conversely, a persisting or rising transcript level may suggest the development of drug resistance or poor compliance with imatinib therapy. If evidence of resistance emerges a switch to an alternative next generation tyrosine kinase inhibitor such as dasatinib or nilotinib should be considered.

The impact of tyrosine kinase inhibitors reaches beyond the 3% of children who carry the Philadelphia chromosome. It provides proof of principle that identification of 'driver' mutations in leukaemia can lead to development of targeted therapies which, when used in combination with existing therapies, can transform the outlook for previously poor prognosis groups.

Immunotherapy

It is well known that eradication of malignant cells is an important role of the immune system. One of the major advantages of sibling or unrelated HSCT over twin-to-twin or autologous HSCT is the so-called graft versus leukaemia effect which results in the new incoming immune system identifying any residual host leukaemic cells as 'foreign' and eliminating them. Other approaches can harness immune-based strategies to augment tumor cell kill without resorting to transplantation. Monoclonal antibodies directed against cell surface antigens with or without a conjugated toxin are now in fairly routine use for many cancers. The most widely used in haematology is rituximab, an anti-CD20 antibody which has greatly improved outcome for many B cell lymphomas. Unfortunately, surface CD20 expression is often weak in ALL, particularly in the higher risk cases that would benefit from this approach. Other more suitable targets include CD19 (XmAb5574), CD22 (epratuzumab, moxetumomab pasudotox), CD52 (alemtuzumab) and occasionally CD33 (gemtuzumab ozogamicin). Effective antibodies against CD19 are now being developed, early attempts were hampered by lack of cytotoxic activity, but improved knowledge of effective antibody engineering has now produced drugs with less rapid internalisation and improved antibody dependent cytotoxicty [19].

A particularly promising and more sophisticated approach is to try and redirect host cytotoxic T cells to kill malignant B cells, this has recently been achieved using a bi-specific antibody, blinatumomab, that engages the B cell antigen CD19 and also the CD3 T cell antigen. This brings the cells into close proximity and stimulates T cell-dependent killing. Encouraging results have been reported in adults with relapsed and refractory ALL [20]; paediatric phase 1 and 2 trials are in progress.

Personalised Molecular Genetics

A huge explosion of information has recently become available on additional genetic abnormalities associated with leukaemia. A number of important poor prognostic mutations such as *IKAROS* gene deletions have been identified [21]. The current challenge is to know how to use this information to modify treatment of individual children. It is unlikely that this genetic information will supersede MRD as it only provides information about intrinsic leukaemia cell biology rather than a global measure of host, leukaemic and drug factors. In addition, the prognostic significance of a genetic marker may depend on many variables. The pseudo-autosomal cytokine receptor-like factor 2 gene, *CRLF2*, provides a very good example of the complexity involved in analyzing the impact of even a single genetic marker. Overexpression of CRLF2 was initially identified as being a very poor prognostic feature amongst children enrolled on COG protocols [22]. Overexpression is usually due to one of two defined genetic lesions, most commonly *CRLF2* is fused to the promoter of the *P2RY8* gene *(CRLF2-P2RY8)*, alternatively it may be fused to the *IGH@* enhancer (*IGH@-CRLF2*). In the COG trials the *IGH@-CRLF2* rearrangement was more frequent in National Cancer Institute high-risk patients of Latin-Hispanic ethnicity and was associated with a poor outcome [22]. European trial groups went on to characterise mutation status in their patients and came to conflicting conclusions. In the AIEOP-BFM trial (Italy, Austria and Germany), where patients were initially screened for high CRLF2 expression followed by mutation analysis, there was a subset of patients with the *CRLF2-P2RY8* translocation who were in the non-HR group by MRD determination but nonetheless did very poorly, suggesting that detection of *CRLF2-P2RY8* could provide additional information over and above MRD status [23]. In the MRC ALL97 trial meanwhile, *CRLF2* rearrangements were shown to have no independent prognostic value and patients had an outcome similar to patients with intermediate risk cytogenetics [23]. Finally, an analysis was carried out of all patients with either translocation in both the AIEOP-BFM and MRC trials to see if treatment protocol influenced outcome [23]. Interestingly, whilst the *CRLF2-P2RY8* patients had similar outcomes on both trials, the *IGH@-CRLF2* group had markedly different outcomes. Amongst the 9 patients with *IGH@-CRLF2* in AIEOP-BFM none relapsed, suggesting it was low-risk, whereas in the UK MRC UKALL97 trial 5/6 patients with the *IGH@-CRLF2* translocation relapsed and subsequently died from disease, confirming the reported association with high-risk disease [23]. This strikingly apparent difference in outcome could be an artefact due to the small number of patients involved. However, it could also be related to use of earlier intensification in the AIEOP-BFM trial protocol or reflect subtle differences in the participants between different national trials. Overall, this illustrates how difficult it will be to incorporate individual genetic lesions into personalised treatment strategies since the outcome may depend on not only the presence or absence of a particular genetic change but also the exact nature of the translocation partner/basepair change, the screening method employed to detect it, the presence of other modifying genetic lesions, the ethnic background of the patient and the exact chemotherapy protocol delivered.

Of course this great increase in genetic information is proving extremely useful in adding to the body of knowledge on leukaemia disease biology and cancer biology in general. For example, use of high-resolution single nucleotide polymorphism arrays along with next-generation sequencing and whole genome sequencing of blasts from childhood ALL samples has provided extensive insight into the clonal evolution of cancer and likely driver mutations for disease progression [24, 25]. In addition, it has helped define new previously unappreciated leukaemia subtypes such as early T cell precursor (ETP) ALL [26]. ETP ALL arises in stem cell like precursors which have recently emigrated from the bone marrow to the thymus. Early reports suggest that the gene expression profile of ETP ALL is closer to that seen in haematopoietic stem cells or acute myeloid leukaemia (AML) than lymphoid leukaemia. Cases often display upregulation of the *FLT3* tyrosine kinase gene, more normally associated with AML, providing a potential novel therapeutic target as FLT3 inhibitors are in widespread use for AML [26]. Other gene-expression profiling (microarray) studies have shown that infant ALL displays many similarities to acute myeloid leukaemia resulting in 'AML-type' chemotherapy blocks being incorporated into the latest infant ALL trials. Finally, these unbiased genome wide approaches may lead to the identification of key players in disease pathology that may become novel therapeutic targets, a particularly important approach for patients with very high risk disease [27]. Such approaches have already identified activating mutations in Janus kinases (JAK) and currently COG are running a phase 1 clinical trial of a JAK inhibitor (ruxolitinib) for relapsed and refractory paediatric tumours.

Is Personalised Therapy Only Realistic in Rich Healthcare Systems?

Although some of the techniques described above are clearly expensive, and remain the preserve of economically rich healthcare systems, it is reassuring that simple risk stratification is very cheap and inexpensive. Effective treatment of ALL in developing counties is often hampered by infectious mortality related to treatment rather than relapse rate. Therefore, the ability to identify very good risk patients who can be spared highly myelosuppressive regimens associated with high rates of infectious mortality should have a significant impact on survival rates. Stratification by age and white cell count remains useful and addition of simple measures of treatment sensitivity such as the 7-day Prednisolone response only require a light microscope. More recently groups have reported that the use of simplified flow cytometry assay after 2 weeks of steroid treatment can reliably identify children with ultra-low-risk disease who could be spared intensive treatment [28].

Future Directions

Childhood ALL has been at the forefront of development of personalised medicine. It is fair to say that many children with ALL now benefit from highly individualised treatment using a multitude of genetic and phenotype based approaches. It is remarkable that such an approach cannot only help to direct treatment in children with adverse features but also be used as a tool to identify and de-escalate therapy in children with good risk features. New advances are being made all the time and are starting to filter through to other areas of haematology and oncology in both paediatric and adult practice. There is no room for complacency however; the treatment of children with refractory and very high risk disease remains difficult, infants fare poorly, and too many children with curable disease still suffer significant disabling treatment-related toxicity. In addition, there is much still to learn about the causes of leukaemia and strategies to prevent its occurrence in the first place. It is hoped that the explosion of high-resolution genetic information, advances in molecular pharmacology, the ability to track the response to treatment using MRD and a better understanding of how to optimally harness the immune system will lead to further improvements in outcome for all patients with malignancy.

References

1 Pui CH, Campana D, Pei D, Bowman WP, Sandlund JT, Kaste SC, Ribeiro RC, Rubnitz JE, Raimondi SC, Onciu M, Coustan-Smith E, Kun LE, Jeha S, Cheng C, Howard SC, Simmons V, Bayles A, Metzger ML, Boyett JM, Leung W, Handgretinger R, Downing JR, Evans WE, Relling MV: Treating childhood acute lymphoblastic leukemia without cranial irradiation. N Engl J Med 2009;360:2730–2741.

2 Hunger SP, Lu X, Devidas M, Camitta BM, Gaynon PS, Winick NJ, Reaman GH, Carroll WL: Improved survival for children and adolescents with acute lymphoblastic leukemia between 1990 and 2005: a report from the children's oncology group. J Clin Oncol 2012;30:1663–1669.

3 Farber S, Diamond LK: Temporary remissions in acute leukemia in children produced by folic acid antagonist, 4-aminopteroyl-glutamic acid. N Engl J Med 1948;238:787–793.

4 Pinkel D: Five-year follow-up of 'total therapy' of childhood lymphocytic leukemia. JAMA 1971;216: 648–652.

5 Halsey C, Buck G, Richards S, Vargha-Khadem F, Hill F, Gibson B: The impact of therapy for childhood acute lymphoblastic leukaemia on intelligence quotients; results of the risk-stratified randomized central nervous system treatment trial MRC UKALL XI. J Hematol Oncol 2011;4:42.

6 Boissel N, Auclerc MF, Lheritier V, Perel Y, Thomas X, Leblanc T, Rousselot P, Cayuela JM, Gabert J, Fegueux N, Piguet C, Huguet-Rigal F, Berthou C, Boiron JM, Pautas C, Michel G, Fiere D, Leverger G, Dombret H, Baruchel A: Should adolescents with acute lymphoblastic leukemia be treated as old children or young adults? Comparison of the French FRALLE-93 and LALA-94 trials. J Clin Oncol 2003; 21:774–780.
7 Moorman AV, Ensor HM, Richards SM, Chilton L, Schwab C, Kinsey SE, Vora A, Mitchell CD, Harrison CJ: Prognostic effect of chromosomal abnormalities in childhood B-cell precursor acute lymphoblastic leukaemia: results from the UK Medical Research Council ALL97/99 randomised trial. Lancet Oncol 2010;11:429–438.
8 Conter V, Bartram CR, Valsecchi MG, et al: Molecular response to treatment redefines all prognostic factors in children and adolescents with B-cell precursor acute lymphoblastic leukemia: results in 3,184 patients of the AIEOP-BFM ALL 2000 study. Blood 2010;115:3206–3214.
9 van der Velden VH, Hochhaus A, Cazzaniga G, Szczepanski T, Gabert J, van Dongen JJ: Detection of minimal residual disease in hematologic malignancies by real-time quantitative PCR: principles, approaches, and laboratory aspects. Leukemia 2003;17: 1013–1034.
10 Cazzaniga G, Valsecchi MG, Gaipa G, Conter V, Biondi A: Defining the correct role of minimal residual disease tests in the management of acute lymphoblastic leukaemia. Br J Haematol 2011;155:45–52.
11 Vora A, Goulden N, Wade R, Mitchell C, Hancock J, Hough R, Rowntree C, Richards S: Treatment reduction for children and young adults with low-risk acute lymphoblastic leukaemia defined by minimal residual disease (UKALL 2003): a randomised controlled trial. Lancet Oncol 2013;14:199–209.
12 Bowman WP, Larsen EL, Devidas M, Linda SB, Blach L, Carroll AJ, Carroll WL, Pullen DJ, Shuster J, Willman CL, Winick N, Camitta BM, Hunger SP, Borowitz MJ: Augmented therapy improves outcome for pediatric high risk acute lymphocytic leukemia: results of Children's Oncology Group trial P9906. Pediatr Blood Cancer 2011;57:569–577.
13 Parker C, Waters R, Leighton C, Hancock J, Sutton R, Moorman AV, Ancliff P, Morgan M, Masurekar A, Goulden N, Green N, Revesz T, Darbyshire P, Love S, Saha V: Effect of mitoxantrone on outcome of children with first relapse of acute lymphoblastic leukaemia (ALL R3): an open-label randomised trial. Lancet 2010;376:2009–2017.
14 Evans WE, Relling MV, Rodman JH, Crom WR, Boyett JM, Pui CH: Conventional compared with individualized chemotherapy for childhood acute lymphoblastic leukemia. N Engl J Med 1998;338:499–505.
15 Relling MV, Gardner EE, Sandborn WJ, Schmiegelow K, Pui CH, Yee SW, Stein CM, Carrillo M, Evans WE, Klein TE: Clinical Pharmacogenetics Implementation Consortium guidelines for thiopurine methyltransferase genotype and thiopurine dosing. Clin Pharmacol Ther 2011;89:387–391.
16 Nersting J, Borst L, Schmiegelow K: Challenges in implementing individualized medicine illustrated by antimetabolite therapy of childhood acute lymphoblastic leukemia. Clin Proteomics 2011;8:8.
17 Schultz KR, Bowman WP, Aledo A, Slayton WB, Sather H, Devidas M, Wang C, Davies SM, Gaynon PS, Trigg M, Rutledge R, Burden L, Jorstad D, Carroll A, Heerema NA, Winick N, Borowitz MJ, Hunger SP, Carroll WL, Camitta B: Improved early event-free survival with imatinib in Philadelphia chromosome-positive acute lymphoblastic leukemia: a children's oncology group study. J Clin Oncol 2009;27:5175–5181.
18 Biondi A, Schrappe M, De Lorenzo P, Castor A, Lucchini G, Gandemer V, Pieters R, Stary J, Escherich G, Campbell M, Li CK, Vora A, Arico M, Rottgers S, Saha V, Valsecchi MG: Imatinib after induction for treatment of children and adolescents with Philadelphia-chromosome-positive acute lymphoblastic leukaemia (EsPhALL): a randomised, open-label, intergroup study. Lancet Oncol 2012;13:936–945.
19 Zalevsky J, Leung IW, Karki S, Chu SY, Zhukovsky EA, Desjarlais JR, Carmichael DF, Lawrence CE: The impact of Fc engineering on an anti-CD19 antibody: increased Fc-gamma-receptor affinity enhances B-cell clearing in nonhuman primates. Blood 2009;113: 3735–3743.
20 Topp MS, Kufer P, Gokbuget N, Goebeler M, Klinger M, Neumann S, Horst HA, Raff T, Viardot A, Schmid M, Stelljes M, Schaich M, Degenhard E, Kohne-Volland R, Bruggemann M, Ottmann O, Pfeifer H, Burmeister T, Nagorsen D, Schmidt M, Lutterbuese R, Reinhardt C, Baeuerle PA, Kneba M, Einsele H, Riethmuller G, Hoelzer D, Zugmaier G, Bargou RC: Targeted therapy with the T-cell-engaging antibody blinatumomab of chemotherapy-refractory minimal residual disease in B-lineage acute lymphoblastic leukemia patients results in high response rate and prolonged leukemia-free survival. J Clin Oncol 2011; 29:2493–2498.
21 Chen IM, Harvey RC, Mullighan CG, Gastier-Foster J, Wharton W, Kang H, Borowitz MJ, Camitta BM, Carroll AJ, Devidas M, Pullen DJ, Payne-Turner D, Tasian SK, Reshmi S, Cottrell CE, Reaman GH, Bowman WP, Carroll WL, Loh ML, Winick NJ, Hunger SP, Willman CL: Outcome modeling with CRLF2, IKZF1, JAK, and minimal residual disease in pediatric acute lymphoblastic leukemia: a Children's Oncology Group study. Blood 2012;119:3512–3522.

22 Harvey RC, Mullighan CG, Chen IM, Wharton W, Mikhail FM, Carroll AJ, Kang H, Liu W, Dobbin KK, Smith MA, Carroll WL, Devidas M, Bowman WP, Camitta BM, Reaman GH, Hunger SP, Downing JR, Willman CL: Rearrangement of CRLF2 is associated with mutation of JAK kinases, alteration of IKZF1, Hispanic/Latino ethnicity, and a poor outcome in pediatric B-progenitor acute lymphoblastic leukemia. Blood 2010;115:5312–5321.
23 Attarbaschi A, Morak M, Cario G, Cazzaniga G, Ensor HM, Te Kronnie T, Bradtke J, Mann G, Vendramini E, Palmi C, Schwab C, Russell LJ, Schrappe M, Conter V, Mitchell CD, Strehl S, Zimmermann M, Potschger U, Harrison CJ, Stanulla M, Panzer-Grumayer R, Haas OA, Moorman AV: Treatment outcome of CRLF2 -rearranged childhood acute lymphoblastic leukaemia: a comparative analysis of the AIEOP-BFM and UK NCRI-CCLG study groups. Br J Haematol 2012;158:772–777.
24 Mullighan CG, Phillips LA, Su X, Ma J, Miller CB, Shurtleff SA, Downing JR: Genomic analysis of the clonal origins of relapsed acute lymphoblastic leukemia. Science 2008;322:1377–1380.
25 Greaves M, Maley CC: Clonal evolution in cancer. Nature 2012;481:306–313.
26 Zhang J, Ding L, Holmfeldt L, et al: The genetic basis of early T-cell precursor acute lymphoblastic leukaemia. Nature 2012;481:157–163.
27 Roberts KG, Morin RD, Zhang J, et al: Genetic alterations activating kinase and cytokine receptor signaling in high-risk acute lymphoblastic leukemia. Cancer Cell 2012;22:153–166.
28 Coustan-Smith E, Ribeiro RC, Stow P, Zhou Y, Pui CH, Rivera GK, Pedrosa F, Campana D: A simplified flow cytometric assay identifies children with acute lymphoblastic leukemia who have a superior clinical outcome. Blood 2006;108:97–102.

Christina Halsey
Institute of Infection, Immunity and Inflammation, College of Medical Veterinary and Life Sciences, Level 3, Glasgow Biomedical Research Centre
University of Glasgow, 120, University Place, Glasgow G12 8TA (UK)
E-Mail chris.halsey@glasgow.ac.uk

Thomas AE, Halsey C (eds): Controversies in Pediatric and Adolescent Hematology.
Pediatr Adolesc Med. Basel, Karger, 2014, vol 17, pp 116–134 (DOI: 10.1159/000350350)

Reduced Intensity Conditioning in Paediatric Haematopoietic Cell Transplantation

Robert Chiesa · Paul Veys

Great Ormond Street Hospital for Children NHS Foundation Trust, London, UK

Abstract

Haematopoietic cell transplantation (HCT) is a recognised curative approach for children and adults affected by malignant and non-malignant haematological disorders. Nevertheless, myeloablative preparative regimens are associated with significant short-term toxicity and long-term sequelae. The principle of a reduced intensity-conditioning (RIC) regimen is to achieve a state of stable donor engraftment at a level sufficient to cure the underlying disease or ameliorate its clinical phenotype, while reducing the complications associated with myeloablative strategies. The use of RIC-HCT has been particularly explored in children with non-malignant diseases and the available data suggest that disorders such as primary immunodeficiencies should be treated with an RIC approach even in the absence of comorbidities. In contrast, the indication for RIC-HCT in children with haematological malignancies is less robust, and this approach should be limited to patients who are clinically unfit for, or have relapsed after, myeloablative HCT. In either setting, RIC regimens have extended the possibility of HCT to patients with pre-transplant comorbidities that would otherwise have precluded them from a conventional transplant procedure. Here, we summarise the current status and future directions of the use of RIC-HCT in paediatric patients.

Copyright © 2014 S. Karger AG, Basel

The field of haematopoietic cell transplantation (HCT) had its firm beginnings in paediatrics with the first successful bone marrow transplant being performed in 1968 in a child with severe combined immune deficiency. Today, more than 15,000 allogeneic HCTs per year are performed worldwide, with around one quarter of those occurring in children suffering from a wide variety of malignant and genetic disorders. There is no doubt that HCT represents one of the most innovative treatments of the last decades, and while the principles of HCT have remained the same, dramatic changes in the details of HCT over the last 40 years have led to significant improvements in outcome. While many children are now cured from otherwise fatal disorders, much work is still required to reduce both acute toxicities, and specifically in children, the long-term side effects of these procedures. The answer to these problems may come from the adult world with the advent of reduced intensity conditioning HCT procedures.

Traditional myeloablative preparation for HCT is associated with a high incidence of transplant-related morbidity and mortality (TRM), as well as long-term sequelae. With the realisation of potential graft-versus-marrow and graft-versus-leukaemia (GvL) responses associated with allogeneic HCT, investigators have explored the use of reduced-intensity conditioning (RIC) prior to HCT in older individuals as well as younger adults with comorbidities, otherwise ineligible for myeloablative procedures. Although there has been a higher incidence of relapse in some cohorts, TRM has been significantly reduced, and over the last 15 years RIC-HCT has become a well-established strategy in adult patients with malignant diseases [1]. Because paediatric patients generally tolerate more intensive transplant approaches, myeloablative regimens have continued to be preferred in childhood malignancies, while RIC has become an attractive option for children with non-malignant diseases particularly those with pre-transplant infections and organ toxicities, both common for instance in children with primary immune deficiency diseases.

Definition of Reduced-Intensity Conditioning Regimens

Compared to fully intensive conditioning regimens, RIC protocols have been traditionally characterised by the following qualities:

- reversible myelosuppression (typically within 28 days) in the absence of stem cell support;
- reduced regimen-related toxicity;
- higher incidence of mixed donor haematopoiesis (mixed chimerism).

In practice, the Third European Group for Blood and Marrow Transplantation (EBMT) workshop on RIC-HCT [2] used one or more of the following criteria to define an RIC regimen:

- total-body irradiation (TBI) ≤200 cGy;
- ≤8 mg/kg total busulfan (BU) dose;
- ≤140 mg/m^2 total melphalan (MEL) dose;
- ≤10 mg/kg total thiotepa dose.

Two general approaches have been used to develop RIC regimens; the terminology may be confusing but RIC protocols may be further subdivided into those with minimal-intensity conditioning (MIC) (fig. 1). RIC protocols still contain drugs capable of targeting stem cells (e.g. BU or MEL), but at a reduced dose compared with conventional myeloablative therapy. RIC regimens require HCT for a rapid haematological recovery and if the graft is rejected, aplasia may occur for up to 28 days. Initial chimerism following RIC-HCT is therefore frequently 100% donor, but may de-

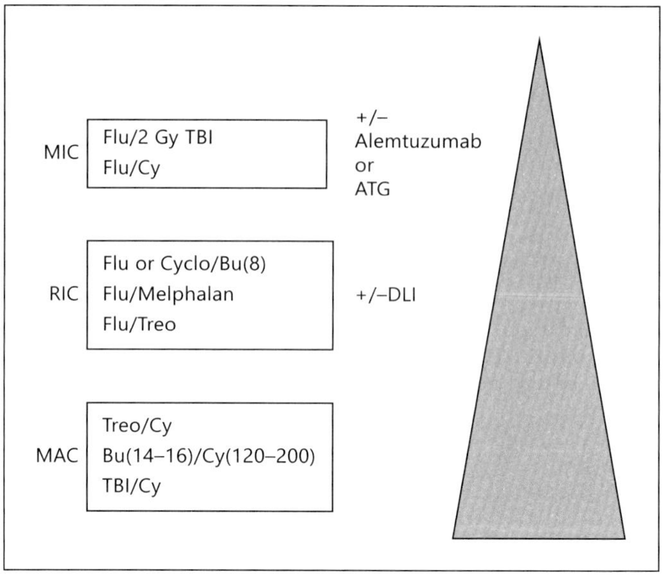

Fig. 1. A hierarchy of commonly used MIC, RIC and MAC regimens in primary immunodeficiency patients; Flu = Fludarabine; Cyclo = cyclophosphamide; BU(8) = busulfan 8 mg/kg; BU(14–16) = busulfan 14–16 mg/kg; Cy(120–200) = cyclophosphamide 120–200 mg/kg; Treo = treosulfan; DLI = donor lymphocyte infusion; ATG = anti-thymocyte globulin. From Bone Marrow Transplant 2008;41: 174, with permission (modified).

cline thereafter in the absence of an adequate graft-versus-marrow effect, as autologous haematopoiesis recovers resulting in mixed chimerism. By contrast, MIC regimens are strictly non-myeloablative and contain only immunosuppressive agents. A truly non-myeloablative/MIC regimen does not eradicate host haematopoiesis and allows relatively rapid autologous haematopoietic recovery without a transplant, but is sufficiently myelosuppressive to enable at least partial donor engraftment to occur post-HCT [3]. In this setting initial chimerism is often mixed.

While stable mixed chimerism in the disease lineage is likely to correct phenotypic expression of certain genetic diseases, patients with haematological malignancies will require full donor engraftment, and if 100% donor chimerism is not achieved or is initially achieved and then lost following RIC/MIC HCT then an enhanced graft-versus-marrow effect will be required to control disease usually involving a rapid tail of immunosuppression and use of donor lymphocyte infusions (DLIs).

Reduced-Intensity Conditioning in Malignant Diseases

Many studies have analysed the use of RIC-HCT in adults affected by malignant haematological diseases, although most of these reports focus on elderly patients undergoing HCT from a matched family donor. However, in the last decade or so the RIC approach has also been tested in younger patients undergoing HCT from alternative donors. Adults affected by haematological malignancies such as acute myeloid leukaemia (AML), chronic myeloid leukaemia (CML), Hodgkin disease (HD) and non-Hodgkin lymphoma have been successfully cured with RIC protocols, confirming the premise that RIC-HCT can minimise TRM in elderly patients, or in those with significant pre-transplant co-morbidities, while exerting a powerful graft-versus-tumor (GvT) effect to cure the disease [4]. A comparison between the RIC and myeloablative conditioning (MAC) strategy in this context has been studied by a few groups, with comparable outcomes [5, 6], although some studies have suggested an increased incidence of disease relapse after RIC-HCT. Since paediatric patients affected by haematological malignancies can generally tolerate high-dose chemo-/radiotherapy protocols better than adults, only a few RIC-HCT studies have been performed in children in this setting. Such reports have been mainly focused on children with haematological malignancies and medically unfit for a myeloablative procedure or children with an indication for a second HCT. Del Toro et al. [7] reported the results of 14 paediatric patients affected by different malignant diseases and treated with a fludarabine (FLU)-based regimen followed by allogeneic HCT. Six patients had been treated for HD (3 children in second complete remission (CR2), 1 child in partial remission (PR) and 2 patients had progressive disease (PD)), one patient had non-Hodgkin lymphoma in PR, 2 patients had neuroblastoma (1 in CR and 1 with PD), 1 patient had Wilms' tumour with PD, 1 patient had CML in the chronic phase, 1 patient had AML in first CR (CR1) and 2 patients were affected by myelodysplastic syndrome manifesting as refractory anaemia. Most patients received BU (≤8 mg/kg)/FLU/anti-thymocyte globulin (ATG), except one child with CML who received BU (8 mg/kg)/FLU/alemtuzumab and one patient with HD who received cyclophosphamide (CY)/FLU/ATG. Graft versus host disease (GvHD) prophylaxis consisted of tacrolimus and mycophenolate mofetil (MMF). The incidence of grade II–IV acute GvHD (aGvHD) and chronic GvHD (cGvHD) was 38 and 0%, respectively. The reported 1-year overall survival (OS) of this study was 78%. This report demonstrated that a high level of sustained donor chimerism and myeloid engraftment can be achieved in children with malignant diseases following RIC-HCT with either a matched family donor or unrelated cord blood donor. In another study, Gómez-Almaguer et al. [8] reported their experience with RIC-HCT in 16 children and adolescents with malignant diseases who received allogeneic HCT from matched sibling donors following a RIC protocol with low dose BU and CY. Thirteen children had acute lymphoblastic leukaemia (ALL) (7 in second remission, 1 in third remission, 1 in first relapse, 3 in second relapse and 1 primarily refractory to therapy), 1 patient had AML and 1 had CML in accelerated phase. GvHD prophylaxis consisted of cyclosporine (CsA) and methotrexate. The incidence of aGvHD and cGvHD was 9.5 and 13%, respectively. In this study the 2-year OS rate was 44%. However, the event-free survival was 47% for high-risk ALL patients. Overall, this regimen was very well tolerated and cost effective as half of the patients received RIC-HCT in an outpatient setting. However, the results of these studies should be interpreted with caution since larger groups of children with homogeneous diagnoses, disease status, uniform cell source and RIC regimens need to be studied.

There are four major disease-specific studies on RIC-HCT in children with haematological malignancies. The first study describes 11 children with very high-risk ALL who were ineligible for standard intensity conditioning, who received a FLU/BU/ATG-based RIC-HCT with GvHD prophylaxis consisting of CsA only [9]. A high degree of donor chimerism was achieved, and 36% of patients achieved remission following such RIC-HCT. Two patients developed grade IV aGvHD. Two of 5 patients surviving more than 100 days developed cGvHD. Overall TRM was high (50%). In the second study at Columbia University Medical Center, 8 children with CD33+ AML in CR1 (n = 5) or CR2 (n = 3) received targeted immunotherapy with gemtuzumab ozogamicin after RIC-HCT during the period of potential minimal residual disease. The RIC regimen consisted of BU (≤8 mg/kg)/FLU±ATG and tacrolimus/MMF used for GvHD prophylaxis. The RIC regimen was well tolerated without any significant morbidity or mortality and the incidence of grade II–IV aGvHD and cGvHD was very low (12.5% each). In this study, the OS was 63%, which is comparable to standard intensity regimens [10]. Claviez et al. [11] reported a small study of 6 children with refractory (n = 4)/relapsed (n = 2) HD who received a RIC protocol consisting of BU (≤8 mg/kg)/FLU±CY. In this high-risk group of patients, 3 of 6 children survived following RIC-HCT. More recently, Corker et al. [12] addressed the efficacy and feasibility of a reduced intensity, treosulfan-based conditioning in infants affected by high-risk ALL with MLL gene rearrangement undergoing HCT. Six children were treated with treosulfan (total dose 36–42 g/m^2) and CY (120 mg/kg) prior to a matched sibling donor bone marrow transplantation (n = 1) or an unrelated umbilical cord blood transplantation (n = 5). Acute GvHD grade ≥2 was observed in 2 children. Primary engraftment occurred in all patients, with 5/6 patients maintaining 100% donor engraftment. Regimen-related toxicity was low, with 1 case of mild veno-occulsive disease (VOD) and 1 septic episode. One patient presented with a bone marrow relapse post-HCT, while the other 5 children were alive and in CR with a median follow-up of 5 years. This regimen proved to be effective and safe in a subgroup of children affected by high-risk disease and historically treated with aggressive preparative regimens such as BU/CY/MEL. Recently, there have been promising data in adult patients with refractory AML undergoing sequential conditioning with fludarabine, cytosine arabinoside, and amsacrine RIC-HCT [13]. The data in children are still very limited but based on 7 children affected by refractory relapsed AML, 2 are surviving disease free, with leukaemia-free survival being closely related to the use of DLI to augment a GvL effect [Sauer M, pers. commun., 2012].

The chimeric state after RIC-HCT provides an ideal platform for adoptive cellular immunotherapy. Donor lymphocyte infusion can be given after RIC-HCT for conversion from mixed to full donor chimerism, as a pre-emptive strategy to prevent leukaemia relapse or for the treatment of haematological malignancies relapsing post-transplant and for conditions such as lymphoproliferative disease. Achievement of remission following DLI depends to a large extent on the underlying disease with best responses demonstrated in the treatment of relapse of CML (70–80%) and, in a more paediatric setting, of juvenile myelomonocytic leukaemia and other myeloproliferative/myelodysplastic disorders and to a lesser extent in Philadelphia-positive (Ph^+) ALL. Data on the use of DLI for relapsed pediatric malignancies after RIC-HCT are limited, but in principle RIC-HCT may allow patients with such diseases who are not fit for conventional intensity conditioning to benefit from immunotherapy with DLI either pre-emptively or in relapse. For the majority of patients, however, the cytoreduction afforded by conventional MAC offers the best platform from which to exert a GvL effect after a primary transplant procedure. However, for patients with myeloid leukaemia, myelodysplastic syndrome and Ph^+ ALL who relapse after a myeloablative HCT having never developed significant GvHD, RIC may enable a second HCT engineered to generate GvH/GvL, within a few months from the first transplantation. This may be a better approach than DLI alone particularly in the setting of acute leukaemia, as the 2nd HCT is likely to reduce disease burden more effectively giving time for GvL effects to work. Raghuram et al. [14] reported long-term survival in 3/6 children with haematological malignancies relapsing after initial myeloablative transplant and likewise Nagler et al. [15] observed disease-free survival in 6/12 mostly adult patients receiving a second non-myeloablative HCT for haematological malignancies. Although the use of DLI to induce GvT and prevent or treat leukaemia relapse is promising, high response rates are still limited to CML and other myeloproliferative diseases and outcome is compromised by the risk of significant GvHD. Recently, more innovative approaches have been pursued to both maximise GvT and minimise GvHD after HCT. Genetic engineering can provide cytotoxic T cells with specific antigenic properties, and such antigen specific T cells can be expanded and administered as adoptive immunotherapy. Both genetically engineered T cell receptors recognising antigens in an MHC-restricted fashion, as well as genetically engineered receptors that include the binding sites of monoclonal antibodies (chimeric antigen receptors or CARs) have been explored in this setting. CAR-transduced cells have been demonstrated to migrate to tumour sites and clinical trials using a CAR against GD2, a receptor expressed on tumour cells of neuroectodermal origin, have been completed in children with neuroblastoma, with no toxicity noted. Pule et al. [16] showed a 50% response rate (including one sustained CR) in children affected by neuroblastoma and treated with Epstein-Barr virus (EBV)-specific cytotoxic lymphocytes engineered to recognise GD2. Clinical trials with genetically engineered T cell receptors and CARs in paediatric patients with ALL (some following reduced intensity HCT) are ongoing and additional protocols are in development for children with lymphoma, medulloblastoma, and glioblastoma multiforme.

Finally, in view of the increased risk of relapse following RIC-HCT, investigators have focused on reduced toxicity HCT by targeting therapy to the marrow and/or disease. Schulz et al. [17] have published results on the use of targeted irradiation to the bone marrow with yttrium-90-labelled anti-CD66 monoclonal antibody in children affected by a variety of malignant and non-malignant diseases. Interestingly 2/5 children affected by relapsed/refractory acute leukaemia and treated with radioimmunotherapy in the context of a fludarabine-based RIC were alive and in CR 30 months after HCT. A paediatric phase I, escalating dose study on the use of radioimmunotherapy prior to HCT is about to open in Great Ormond Street Hospital (GOSH), London.

Reduced Intensity Conditioning in Primary Immune Deficiencies

The use of RIC-HCT has been studied more extensively in children affected by non-malignant diseases, with a particular focus on primary immunodeficiencies (PID) [18]. In fact, most of these disorders can be clinically cured with the achievement of a mixed donor stem cell engraftment, therefore providing a strong rationale for the choice of RIC protocols in this context. Importantly, the use of conditioning regimens at reduced intensity may reduce both short- and long-term toxicities/sequelae after stem cell transplant, making this strategy particularly appropriate in childhood. Different combinations of drugs have been studied, showing that the use of RIC-HCT for the treatment of paediatric non-malignant diseases is safe and effective.

The GOSH in London was the first Institution to report the results on the use of fludarabine and MEL with alemtuzumab in children affected by PID. In spite of significant co-morbidities at the time of transplant, 7/8 children were alive and engrafted 8–17 months post-HCT [19]. These preliminary results have been recently updated, describing 113 children with PID who underwent RIC-HCT between 1998 and 2006. A significant proportion of children had severe co-morbidities prior to HCT, including previous mechanical ventilation (n = 12), liver or renal impairment (n = 8) or total parental nutrition-dependent enteropathy (n = 8). Most children (93/113) received a RIC protocol with alemtuzumab 1 mg/kg, fludarabine 150 mg/m^2 and MEL 140 mg/m^2, while 20 patients underwent a MIC HCT. The overall survival was high (OS = 82%, median follow-up of 2.9 years), and 81% of children achieved a stable donor engraftment, while 12% of patients had or were likely to require additional procedures such as a second HCT, marrow infusion, peripheral stem cell top up or gene therapy [Rao K, pers. commun., 2012].

Although there are no randomised trials comparing RIC versus MAC HCT in primary immunodeficiencies, the GOSH group has retrospectively compared their results in children with PID transplanted from unrelated donors using fludarabine, MEL and alemtuzumab and myeloablative HCT from an earlier time cohort. This study demonstrated a reduced mortality in the RIC group (2/33 RIC versus 4/19 MAC, $p < 0.01$) [20] with an improved OS, and a better survival in children with non-SCID immunodeficiencies. The incidence of acute GvHD was not different between the two groups and, although the immune reconstitution after transplant was comparable, there was a trend towards an increased risk of viral infections and/or reactivations (cytomegalovirus, EBV, adenovirus) in children treated with a RIC protocol

(29% in the RIC group versus 21% following MAC, $p = 0.02$). As predicted, there was an increased incidence of mixed chimerism (MC) after RIC-HCT compared to MAC HCT (45% MC of which 13% had a low-level of donor engraftment in the RIC group, versus 36% MC and 0% with low-level donor engraftment in the MAC group); however, with withdrawal of the immunosuppression, mixed chimerism after RIC appeared to stabilise or move towards full donor engraftment.

The incidence of EBV reactivation after RIC-HCT seems to be higher; the increased rate of EBV viraemia is probably due to the profound immunosuppression that follows RIC-HCT, as well as to the incomplete ablation of recipient-derived B lymphocytes. Nevertheless, the association of alemtuzumab, fludarabine, MEL and rituximab and/or the use of EBV specific cytotoxic T-lymphocytes proved to cure all 8 patients with EBV-driven lympho-proliferative disease complicating PID and immunodysregulatory syndromes [21]. This and other data suggests that EBV monitoring by PCR and pre-emptive treatment (mainly rituximab), can overcome complications associated with EBV viraemia following reduced intensity conditioning HCT. In a similar fashion, a high incidence of CMV reactivation following fludarabine, MEL and alemtuzumab RIC-HCT has been described in adult patients.

In 2005 Shenoy et al. [22] described the use of fludarabine/MEL-prior to HCT in 16 patients with non-malignant disorders. Alemtuzumab was given early pre HCT (from day –21 to day –19) at a dose of 33 or 48 mg. The stem cell source was sibling bone marrow (BM) (n = 5), sibling peripheral blood (PB) (n = 5), unrelated BM (n = 3), and unrelated cord blood (CB) (n = 3). All 14 evaluable patients achieved complete or high level (>50%) donor engraftment in myeloid and lymphoid cell lineages, suggesting that lower doses of alemtuzumab or its early administration may improve donor chimerism in the HLA-matched setting.

The benefit from fludarabine, MEL and alemtuzumab RIC-HCT is most evident in children aged >1 year, since children with SCID below 1 year experienced high TRM (28%) in the London series [GOSH, pers. obs.]. Occasionally, very young patients seem to develop a fatal 'MEL shock' syndrome with significant capillary leak syndrome within hours of receiving MEL although the mechanism of this is not clear. Therefore, an alternative RIC or MIC protocol (e.g. fludarabine and treosulfan, see below) might be advisable for this group of patients. As mentioned above, Schulz et al. [17] have reported their results on RIC-HCT with the combination of fludarabine, MEL and radiolabeled monoclonal antibodies in children with PID [17]. Twelve children with PID underwent HCT from a matched unrelated donor (MUD) or mismatched family donor (n = 8), matched family donor (MFD) (n = 2) or haploidentical donor (n = 2) after conditioning with mostly fludarabine (160 mg/m^2), MEL (70–140 mg/kg) (n = 9/12) and an anti-CD66 monoclonal antibody conjugated with the radioisotope yttrium-90 (^{90}Y-anti-CD66). CD66 is an antigen highly expressed on normal myeloid precursors, and anti-CD66 antibody has been utilised to target radioimmunotherapy in adults with malignancies, achieving positive results in terms of engraftment and toxicity. In this group of children with PID the median dose of irradiation delivered to the bone marrow was 17 Gy (range 16–20 Gy). Eleven patients engrafted, while 1 patient rejected the graft after a haploidentical HCT and eventually died of adenovirus pneumonia. Nine patients achieved 100% donor engraftment at last follow-up (13–49 months), while 2/12 children experienced mixed chimerism. Regimen-related toxicity was low and 10/12 children were alive and disease-free at the last follow-up. These results show that radioimmunotherapy is effective in achieving myeloablation with low additional toxicity when used in combination with RIC in young children affected by PID.

The combination of fludarabine and high-dose BU has progressively replaced the standard myeloablative combination of BU and cyclophosphamide in the majority of transplant centres, due to the increased transplant-related toxicity of the latter strategy, which includes VOD and severe mucositis. A reduced dose of BU associated with fludarabine has also been used as a RIC protocol in children and adults with malignant and non-malignant diseases undergoing HCT. Jacobsohn et al. [23] described the outcome of RIC-HCT in patients with non-malignant diseases using a protocol with fludarabine, low-dose BU and ATG. Six children with PID received a matched sibling donor (MSD) peripheral blood stem cell (PBSC) (n = 2), MUD PBSC (n = 2) and unrelated CB (n = 2) HCT. Patients received fludarabine (180 mg/m^2) and intravenous BU (6.4 mg/kg in 8 doses) on days –5 to –4 or pharmokinetic monitoring to achieve an area under the curve (AUC) of 3,800–4,200 μmol × min with single daily dosing of intravenous BU. Two children with X-linked hyper-IgM syndrome were clinically cured, off intravenous Ig supplementation, and with reversal of their cholangiopathy: 1 patient achieved full donor and one 30% donor engraftment. One patient with X-linked lymphoproliferative disease was also alive and well at the last follow-up with 98% donor engraftment. One child with SCID was too early to evaluate and 2 patients, one with chronic granulomatous disease (CGD) and one with Omenn's syndrome died within 3 months of HCT. There were low rates of acute or chronic GvHD in evaluable patients.

A similar experience has been described by Dennison et al. [24]: 6 children with PID were treated with a combination of fludarabine (150 mg/kg), low-dose intravenous BU (7.8 mg/kg, once daily) and ATG prior to HCT with a MSD (5 cases) or MFD (1 case). All children engrafted, with 4/6 patients achieving mixed chimerism and 2/6 children experiencing full donor engraftment. Transplant-related morbidity was low and all children were alive and clinically cured at the last follow-up.

Horn et al. [25] also reported the use of fludarabine, low-dose BU and ATG in 6 children with PID: intravenous BU was given targeting continuous steady state concentration of 600 ng/ml, while fludarabine was given at a total dose of 160 mg/m^2 and rabbit ATG at a dose of 0.5 mg/kg/day on day –4 and 2.5 mg/kg on days –3 to –1 (total dose 8 mg/kg). Three children achieved >95% donor chimerism and 3 had mixed chimerism. One patient with Wiskott-Aldrich syndrome (WAS) died of CMV pneumonitis, while the others were alive and disease-free at the last follow-up. Interestingly, there were 13 other non-PID patients included in the study and mixed chimerism seemed to be more common with bone marrow as a stem cell source, while graft rejection was more common in patients receiving mismatched grafts. Four patients experienced graft failure, all underwent second HCT and 3/4 are alive and disease-free, showing how a second stem cell transplant after failed first RIC-HCT is frequently successful. Further studies may establish an AUC for intravenous BU that is specifically tailored to different diseases, donor type and stem cell source, in order to achieve lineage specific donor engraftment with minimum acute and long-term morbidity. A recent and successful example of this kind of PK approach is provided by Gungor et al. [26] in the treatment of CGD (see below).

Historically, conditioning regimens prior to HCT have been based on the combination of alkylators such as BU, cyclophosphamide or MEL, but side effects such as severe mucosal damage, VOD or cardio-toxicity have led to explore the use of alternative drugs in order to improve the outcome after HCT, whilst minimising its morbidity. Treosulfan (L-threitol-1,4-bis-methanesulphonate) is the pro-drug of L-diepoxybutane, an alkylating drug with myeloablative and immunosuppressive properties.

Results on treosulfan-based conditioning protocols prior to HCT in adults affected by malignant diseases have demonstrated a high success rate with a lower incidence of regimen-related toxicity such as VOD when compared to BU. Early studies in adults have shown a linear pharmacokinetics of treosulfan up to the clinically effective dose of 42 g/m^2.

Eighteen patients with PID with a mean age <1 year underwent HCT, with a variety of donors and stem cell sources, using treosulfan 14 g/m^2 × 3 days, fludarabine 30 mg/m^2 × 5 days and alemtuzumab (n = 14) or ATG (n = 2) [27]. One patient received cyclophosphamide 50 mg/m^2 × 4 days and ATG. Thirteen patients achieved 100% donor chimerism which remained stable in 10/13 patients. Three children achieved stable mixed chimerism (90–99% donor, n = 2; 30% donor in peripheral blood, but 80% donor in T cells, n = 1) which was sufficient to cure the underlying disease. Two patients achieved low-level donor engraftment (<50%) and are under consideration for a second HCT. Toxicity was tolerable, particularly given such a young group of patients, and may be preferable to the combination of fludarabine, MEL and alemtuzumab in this cohort.

Recently, the UK experience of a treosulfan-based preparative regimen for HCT in children with PID has been published [28]. Forty patients were given a combination of treosulfan (36–42 g/m^2), fludarabine (150 mg/m^2) and alemtuzumab (n = 35) or ATG (n = 3) prior to their HCT. Children underwent an HCT from an unrelated donor (n = 30), MFD (n = 8), MSD (n = 1) or haploidentical donor (n = 1). The majority of the patients (38/40) achieved donor stem cell engraftment, while 2 patients rejected their graft. Twenty-four children (54%) presented full donor engraftment in all cell lineages, while 13 patients achieved mixed chimerism. The majority of patients with mixed chimerism had a high level (≥95%) of donor engraftment in the T cell compartment (n = 11/13), with complete resolution of the disease phenotype. Interestingly, when compared to a similar group of children affected by PID but treated with a combination of treosulfan and cyclophosphamide, patients given fludarabine and treosulfan had a significantly better T cell donor engraftment ($p = 0.038$).

Minimal Intensity Conditioning Protocols for PID

The Seattle group pioneered a MIC protocol prior to HCT in patients (12 children and 2 adults) with PID and coexisting infections, organ toxicity or other factors precluding a more intensive conditioning regimen [29]. Most patients received fludarabine (90 mg/m^2) and low dose TBI (200 cGy) as preparative regimen and all patients received HLA-matched grafts with GvHD prophylaxis consisting of CsA and MMF. No in vivo T cell depletion (ATG or alemtuzumab) was given. Thirteen patients achieved either mixed (n = 5) or full (n = 8) donor chimerism, while one child rejected the graft. Overall survival at 3 years was 62% with a TRM of 23%. However, the incidence of GvHD was high, with 11/14 patients developing mostly grade II acute GvHD and 8 patients developed extensive chronic GvHD, probably due to the use of peripheral blood as the stem cell source and the omission of in vivo T cell depletion. This strategy was associated with a lower incidence of viral infections/reactivations (particularly EBV) compared to RIC regimens with in vivo T cell depletion; however, the high incidence of chronic GvHD would be a limitation to a wider use of this conditioning regimen in children affected by non-malignant disorders.

The GOSH group has adopted a MIC protocol combining the use of fludarabine ($30\ mg/m^2 \times 5$ day, from day –8 to –4) and low-dose cyclophosphamide ($300\ mg/m^2/day \times 4$ days, from day –7 to –4) with two rat anti-CD45 monoclonal antibodies to provide additional myelosuppression and in vivo T cell depletion (alemtuzumab) [30]. Children enrolled in this trial were at high risk of transplant-related morbidity even with RIC protocols due to severe pre-existing organ toxicity, age <1 year, or the presence of DNA/telomere repair disorders. A total of 16 children underwent a MIC HCT from MSD (5), MUD (9) or MMUD (2). The preparative regimen was well tolerated with only 2 patients experiencing grade 3 toxicity (NCI criteria). Six of 16 patients (38%) developed significant acute GvHD (3 children with grade II skin and 3 children with grade III skin/gut GvHD), while 5 children (31%) developed chronic GvHD (limited in 3 and extensive in 2) which resolved in all cases. Not surprisingly, the incidence of GvHD was reduced when BM was used as a stem cell source (2/10 BM recipients compared to 4/4 PBSC recipients developed acute GvHD > grade II). Similarly, the incidence of chronic GvHD was lower in recipients of BM (2/10) as compared to PBSC (3/4). One patient had graft failure with autologous reconstitution, while one child who received a mismatched unrelated cord blood transplant (UCBT) engrafted with stable mixed chimerism. Analysis of chimerism showed that amongst 15 engrafted patients, 6 achieved full donor engraftment, while 5 patients experienced stable high-level mixed chimerism in all cell lineages (57–93%). One patient underwent a second HCT due to very low level donor engraftment. At a median of 37 months post-transplant 13/16 children in this high-risk cohort of patients were alive and cured from their underlying disease. Patients affected by SCID and aged <1 year seemed to have a particular benefit from this MIC HCT protocol.

Source of Stem Cells

The use of PBSCs as opposed to BM in RIC protocols appears to be associated with improved donor engraftment in children affected by PID, but at the cost of an increased incidence of GvHD; in this context, survival appears to be equivalent in the two groups. An unpublished study from GOSH [Rao K, pers. commun., 2011] has recently examined cell lineage-specific chimerism and long-term outcome by donor type and stem cell source in 146 children undergoing HCT after fludarabine and MEL-based conditioning for mostly PID. Stem cell donors were MUD (n = 66), MMUD (n = 45), MSD (n = 17) and family donors (n = 21). Stem cell source was BM (n = 108) or PBSC (n = 41). Overall survival was excellent at 74% (median follow-up 7.4 years), irrespective of stem cell source or donor type. When bone marrow was used as stem cell source there was a higher incidence of rejection (14%) and of very low level (<10%) myeloid engraftment (20% children in the BM group, as opposed to 5% children in the PBSC group). This was particularly evident in the MSD (44% rejection) and MMUD (14% rejection) cohorts. Of note, event-free survival was dismal (21%) in patients with very low level mixed donor chimerism. With the use of PBSC, 95% of children achieved full donor engraftment or high level mixed chimerism. With matched donors, GvHD was equivalent in the BM and PBSC groups. Children undergoing MMUD HCT experienced a higher incidence of acute and chronic GvHD with PBSC (50% grade III and IV acute GVHD, 50% chronic GVHD). Based on these results GOSH recommends the use of PBSC with alemtuzumab, fludarabine and MEL in the MUD setting, but is currently testing the use of CD34+ cell selection (Clinimacs – Miltenyi) from mismatched unrelated donors, with add-back of 3×10^8 CD3+ cells/kg to see whether the excellent engraftment rate of PBSC can be maintained with a GvHD incidence equivalent to the use of BM.

The balance between host versus graft and graft versus host reactions is based on the complex interactions of different stem cell sources with disease type, preparative regimen, in vivo T cell depletion, graft quality (CD34+, CD3+, NK – KIR (natural killer – killer-cell immunoglobulin-like receptor) alloreactivity) and post-transplant immunosuppression; this needs to be more finely balanced in RIC rather than MAC HCT.

There is a limited experience with the use of UCB and RIC in PID. Bradley et al. [31] reported the outcome of 21 children and young adults (median age 9 years) with malignant (n = 14) and non-malignant diseases (n = 7) who underwent a HCT after RIC/MIC regimens. Five patients (2 haemophagocytic lymphohistiocytosis (HLH), 2 SCID and 1 WAS) received 4–6/6 HLA-matched unrelated UCB HCT following MIC conditioning with fludarabine, cyclophosphamide and ATG. Children affected by HLH also received etoposide, but both rejected their graft. Two of the 3 remaining patients died of viral pneumonitis and GvHD-related complications. GOSH have transplanted 3 patients with PID using a MIC protocol: only 1 child survived, while 1 patient died of disseminated cryptosporidiosis and 1 patient of idiopathic pneumonitis [Rao, pers. commun., 2008]. On the basis of limited available literature and personal experience, the use of MIC prior to unrelated UCB HCT does not appear to offer an improved survival in patients with PID.

Recently, Morio et al. [32] published their data on the use of unrelated UCB HCT in 88 children with PID: patients would receive MAC (n = 43), RIC (n = 31) or no conditioning (n = 14) prior to transplant. Children treated with RIC received a variety of preparative regimens including fludarabine and MEL ± low-dose TBI, fludarabine and BU, and fludarabine and low-dose TBI. There was no difference in the incidence of myeloid recovery between the MAC and RIC groups (84 vs. 87% at day +100) and no difference was observed in platelet recovery. The RIC strategy was associated with a reduced mortality as opposed to the MAC group ($p = 0.017$): 87% of children on the RIC regimen and 66% on the MAC regimen were alive at the last follow-up. RIC was chosen mostly for patients with SCID and CGD, with excellent survival rates: 17/18 SCID patients and 3/4 CGD patients remain alive. Interestingly, 8 of 9 patients with PID who underwent UCB HCT following conditioning with treosulfan and fludarabine are alive and well [28].

Altogether, these results suggest that unlike the use of MIC protocols, the combination of RIC and UCB HCT is an attractive approach to HCT in PID.

RIC-HCT in Specific PID Diseases

Chronic Granulomatous Disease

Horwitz et al. [33] published their data on the use of MIC HCT followed by donor lymphocyte infusions (DLI) in 10 patients affected by CGD. The immunosuppressive preparative regimen consisted of cyclophosphamide (120 mg/kg), fludarabine (125 mg/m^2) and ATG, followed by infusion of CD34+ selected peripheral blood stem cells from matched sibling donors. Donor lymphocyte infusions were given at intervals of 30 or more days to increase the level of donor chimerism. After a median follow-up of 17 months, 8/10 patients achieved a level of myeloid engraftment (ranging from 33 to 100%) that should provide normal host immunity. Two patients rejected their graft. Three patients experienced significant acute GHVD, one of whom subsequently had extensive chronic GvHD. Seven patients were alive at the last follow-up: 2 patients died of transplant-related toxicity, while 1 patient died after second stem cell transplantation.

Recently, Gungor et al. [26] updated their data on the use of targeted, low-dose intravenous BU, fludarabine (180 mg/m^2) and in vivo T cell depletion (ATG or alemtuzumab) in 30 high-risk paediatric and adult patients with CGD [24]. BU was infused at 50–65% of the myeloablative dose in adults (6.4–12 mg/kg), while children received an adjusted dose of BU with a targeted cumulative AUC of 45–65 mg/l × h. The majority of the patients were affected by chronic or life-threatening infections and/or inflammatory complications (colitis). Stem cell donors were: matched sibling/related donors (n = 14), MUD (n = 11) and MMUD (n = 5). Bone marrow was the preferred stem cell source. Twenty-eight patients achieved donor engraftment, while 2/30 patients with a low cumulative BU exposure (AUC ≤45 mg/l × h) presented graft rejection with autologous reconstitution and received a second HCT. At last follow-up 28 patients were alive, with good myeloid engraftment (range 95–100%) and cured of the original immunodeficiency. This RIC strategy proved to be effective and well tolerated in both children and adults with CGD and BU dose adjustment was regarded to be of major importance to prevent rejection.

Wiskott-Aldrich Syndrome

The use of RIC-HCT in WAS might be hazardous, since mixed donor chimerism post-transplant might be associated with an increased risk of autoimmunity in this specific condition. Nevertheless, patients affected by WAS and aged >5 years, who have accumulated more co-morbidities generally have a dismal outcome after MAC-HCT, and RIC-HCT may offer an advantage in this context. Investigators in London have studied the use of RIC-HCT in WAS: between 1995 and 2007, 17 children with WAS (median age 27 months) underwent MSD (n = 5) or UD HCT (n = 12). Six patients received a MAC (BU/cyclophosphamide), while RIC-HCT was used in 11 children: treosulfan/fludarabine (n = 5) or fludarabine/MEL (n = 6). Amongst the 11 patients receiving RIC, the donor source was MUD (n = 10) and MMUD (n = 1). Eight children received BM and 3 patients PBSCs. Results in this group were particularly good, since all patients survived with a median follow-up of 4 years. Five of the 17 patients had mixed chimerism all following UD-HCT: 1 patient following MAC UD-HCT, and 4/11children (36%) after RIC UD-HCT. Only 1 of these patients with mixed donor engraftment has developed autoimmune disease so far. Three subsequent children underwent UD HCT with RIC with reduced alemtuzumab (0.6 mg/kg total dose day –8 to day –6), and all achieved 100% donor chimerism with only 1 patient experiencing grade II acute GvHD. Interestingly, 3/4 patients with mixed donor chimerism developed acute GvHD > grade II, as opposed to 3/15 with full donor chimerism ($p < 0.05$). The comparative incidence of mixed chimerism following MAC-HCT in other studies is 28% [34] and 38% [35]. RIC-HCT may be indicated for UD-HCT in WAS, particularly in older children with co-morbidities; nevertheless, some graft-versus-marrow effect is essential to achieve 100% donor engraftment in all patients.

Haemophagocytic Lymphohistiocytosis
Children affected by HLH frequently have significant pre-transplant co-morbidities and require intensive cardio-respiratory support pre-HCT. Such toxicities result in a high TRM with conventional myeloablative protocols, mostly due to non-infectious pulmonary toxicity and VOD. Therefore, the use of RIC has been explored in HLH: 25 consecutive patients with primary HLH underwent RIC-HCT in London, using MUD (n = 8), MMUD (n = 11), MFD (n = 2), and haploidentical (n = 4) donors. Most children received a combination of fludarabine 150 mg/m^2, MEL 140 mg/m^2 and alemtuzumab 1 mg/kg prior to the transplant. Following RIC-HCT, 21/25 (84%) patients were alive and in complete remission: these data compare positively with historical data, especially for children undergoing HCT from a mismatched donor. In the RIC group, 7 of 8 patients (87%) undergoing MUD HCT and 9 of 11 (82%) children undergoing MMUD HCT are alive and in complete remission, as opposed to corresponding figures of 70 and 54% when a myeloablative HCT is used (HLH 94 study).

The London data were confirmed by a study published in 2010 by Marsh et al. [36], who reported the results of 26 children with HLH undergoing a fludarabine/MEL/alemtuzumab conditioned HCT. The authors noted a significant improvement in 3-year OS of patients receiving RIC-HCT (OS = 92%), compared to patients receiving a MAC-HCT in the same institution (OS = 43%). Notably, there were no deaths or cases of VOD prior to day +100 in the RIC group. Nevertheless, there was a high incidence of mixed donor engraftment in the RIC group, occurring in 65% of children and many patients received DLI and/or stem cell boost to stabilise or increase the donor chimerism.

The results of these studies support the use of RIC-HCT in children affected by HLH.

Leucocyte Adhesion Deficiency
Qasim et al. [37] published the HCT experience for 36 children with leucocyte adhesion deficiency treated at 14 centres worldwide between 1993 and 2007: with a median follow-up of 62 months, the overall survival was 75%. Twenty-eight patients underwent MAC HCT, while the remaining 8 children underwent RIC-HCT. Survival after MFD and UD transplants was similar, with 11/14 MFD and 12/14 UD recipients surviving; TRM was more significant after haplo-identical HCT, where 4/8 patients died. Full donor chimerism was achieved in 17 of the survivors, mixed multi-lineage chimerism in 7 patients, and mononuclear cell-restricted chimerism in a further 3 cases. Transplant-related mortality included pneumonitis (n = 2), infection (n = 5), VOD (n = 3) and malignancy (n = 1) and all patients had received MAC HCT. Overall, the use of an RIC strategy appeared to be associated with reduced toxicity, with all 8 patients surviving and although 2 patients have low level donor engraftment, they have not required a 2nd transplant to date.

Reduced Intensity Conditioning in Haemoglobinopathies

Although the survival and quality of life of patients with haemoglobinopathies such as thalassaemia or sickle cell disease has significantly improved with the optimisation of blood transfusion regimens, iron chelation therapy and overall supportive care, allogeneic HCT remains the only curative option. The experience from the transplantation of these patients indicates that stable mixed haematopoietic chimerism with a percentage of donor engraftment as low as 20–30% is sufficient to cure the disease phenotype, therefore raising the possibility that RIC regimens could be used in this setting. Nevertheless, graft failure/graft rejection is already a common complication in the context of a myeloablative conditioning regimen, occurring in 5–30% patients, so an RIC approach carries an even higher risk of graft loss. This was confirmed with one of the first paediatric studies published by Iannone et al. [38], who reported the results on the use of an MIC approach (fludarabine and TBI 2 Gy) in 7 children affected by haemoglobinopathies (sickle cell disease = 6, thalassaemia = 1) undergoing a MSD HCT. Six patients presented a transient donor engraftment but eventually rejected the graft when the immunosuppression was tailed. Although this regimen proved to be minimally toxic, it was not sufficient to achieve a state of immunological tolerance between the stem cell donor and the recipient and prevent graft failure. More recently, a reduced toxicity conditioning regimen consisting on treosulfan, fludarabine and thiotepa, has been successfully used in 60 patients (48 children and 12 adults) affected by thalassaemia [39]; the cumulative incidence of graft failure and TRM was low (9% and 7%, respectively), as well as the incidence of aGvHD (cumulative incidence of grade II–IV aGvHD = 14%). The 5-year probability of survival and thalassaemia-free survival was 93 and 84%. This treosulfan-based conditioning regimen proved to be safe and effective for thalassemia patients given allogeneic HCT, and represents a valid alternative to standard BU-based preparative regimens.

Fertility and Late Effects

One major drive for performing RIC-HCT in children is the reduction of long-term complications associated with MAC-HCT such as growth failure, gonadal failure and secondary malignancies. Nevertheless, the true incidence of late effects following RIC in children with PID awaits well-planned and well-executed follow-up studies as the first cohorts of survivors approach adulthood. Intact fertility and uncomplicated pregnancies have been reported in dogs with canine leucocyte adhesion deficiency following MIC HCT. There have been several reports of successful pregnancies in adults treated with fludarabine, MEL and alemtuzumab or fludarabine, BU and ATG RIC protocols for malignancies; 2 adult patients with CGD fathered children after fludarabine, low-dose BU and ATG; however, the impact of the same drugs on the paediatric gonadal and endocrine systems may be very different and this needs to be addressed in future studies.

Conclusions

While there are no randomised studies comparing RIC-HCT with conventional myeloablative regimens in children, there are sufficient data to indicate that RIC-HCT may have an important role in treating children with PID and HLH; unlike more standard approaches, such regimens can be used without severe toxicity in patients with pre-transplant infections or severe pulmonary or hepatic disease.

Accordingly, RIC has extended the role of allogeneic transplantation to many patients who until recently were considered ineligible for this procedure. RIC-HCT is associated with an increased incidence of mixed donor chimerism and graft rejection compared to fully myeloablative HCT, and while mixed donor engraftment is likely to correct the phenotypic expression of most children with PID, the use of DLI to increase donor chimerism or second HCT may be required in some cases.

It is difficult to make specific recommendations as to which RIC protocol should be used and in which disease and with which donor. As a generalisation the combination of alemtuzumab, fludarabine and MEL is applicable to children aged >1 year undergoing unrelated HCT for immunodeficiency disorders with the greatest benefit realised in T cell deficiencies and HLH. If the donor is fully matched then peripheral blood is the preferred stem cell source. Compared to other RIC protocols the combination of fludarabine and MEL is likely to be associated with the least long-term side effects. The outcome of procedures following treosulfan and fludarabine or reduced BU and fludarabine is likely to be equivalent. Further preference may be guided by the differing incidence of late effects between the two protocols; such studies are urgently required.

The use of RIC protocols in combination with matched sibling donors requires further analysis and in particular the role of in vivo T cell depletion in this context needs to be defined. The role of RIC-HCT is less standardised in children with haematological malignancies and there is a need for randomised, well-controlled clinical trials in selected disease groups. At present, RIC protocols are more suitable in patients affected by diseases more susceptible to a GvL effect such as CML, juvenile myelomonocytic leukaemia and other myelodysplastic/myeloproliferative syndromes. RIC-HCT can also be considered in children with significant pre HCT co-morbidities or in those who are eligible for a second transplant procedure after leukaemia relapse.

Immune-based therapies like DLI represent an approach that could be extensively integrated into current RIC regimens, where the therapeutic strategy relies primarily on the promotion of a GvT effect.

Significant progress in scientific discovery and biotechnology has led to the development of novel cellular/gene strategies with the aim to maximise the anti-tumour immune responses and reduce immune complications of transplantation. A combination of reduced intensity conditioning regimen and post-transplant tumour-specific immunotherapy could improve the safety, specificity and success of allogeneic HCT in children affected by haematological malignancies.

References

1 Barrett AJ, Savani BN: Stem cell transplantation with reduced-intensity conditioning regimens: a review of ten years' experience with new transplant concepts and new therapeutic agents. Leukemia 2006;20: 1661–1672.

2 Bacigalupo A: Third EBMT/AMGEN Workshop on reduced-intensity conditioning allogeneic haemopoietic stem cell transplants (RIC-HSCT), and panel consensus. Bone Marrow Transplant 2004;33:691–696.

3 Giralt S, Estey E, Albitar M, et al: Engraftment of allogeneic hematopoietic progenitor cells with purine analog-containing chemotherapy: harnessing graft-versus-leukemia without myeloablative therapy. Blood 1997;89:4531–4536.

4 Champlin R, et al: Harnessing graft-versus-malignancy: non-myeloablative preparative regimens for allogeneic haematopoietic transplantation, an evolving strategy for adoptive immunotherapy. Br J Haematol 2000;111:18–29.

5 Crawley C, et al: Reduced-intensity conditioning for myeloma: lower nonrelapse mortality but higher relapse rates compared with myeloablative conditioning. Blood 2007;109:3588–3594.

6 Crawley C, et al: Outcomes of reduced-intensity transplantation for chronic myeloid leukemia: an analysis of prognostic factors from the Chronic Leukemia Working Party of the EBMT. Blood 2005;106: 2969–2976.

7 Del Toro G, et al: A pilot study of reduced intensity conditioning and allogeneic stem cell transplantation from unrelated cord blood and matched family donors in children and adolescent recipients. Bone Marrow Transplant 2004;33:613–622.

8 Gómez-Almaguer D, et al: Reduced-intensity stem cell transplantation in children and adolescents: the Mexican experience. Biol Blood Marrow Transplant 2003;9:157–161.

9 Duerst R, et al: Efficacy of RIC with FLU-BU-ATG and allogeneic hematopoietic stem cell transplantation for pediatric ALL. Blood 2004;104:2314 (abstract).

10 Roman E, et al: Preliminary results of the safety of immunotherapy with gemtuzumab ozogamicin following reduced intensity allogeneic stem cell transplant in children with CD33+ acute myeloid leukemia. Clin Cancer Res 2005;11:7164s–7170s.

11 Claviez A, et al: Allogeneic peripheral blood stem cell transplantation following fludarabine-based conditioning in six children with advanced Hodgkin's disease. Ann Hematol 2004;83:237–241.

12 Corker E, Astwood E, Williams J, Vora A: Treosulphan-based radiation-free myeloablative conditioning for allogeneic transplant in infant acute lymphoblastic leukaemia. Br J Haematol 2012;159:104–106.

13 Saure C, et al: Upfront allogeneic blood stem cell transplantation for patients with high-risk myelodysplastic syndrome or secondary acute myeloid leukemia using a FLAMSA-based high-dose sequential conditioning regimen. Biol Blood Marrow Transplant 2012;18:466–472.

14 Raghuram C, et al: Reduced-intensity conditioning in first and second allograft in children without immunodeficiency: experience of three British transplant centres. Bone Marrow Transplant 2004; 33(suppl 1):s48.

15 Nagler A, Or R, Naparstek E, Varadi G, Slavin S: Second allogeneic stem cell transplantation using nonmyeloablative conditioning for patients who relapsed or developed secondary malignancies following autologous transplantation. Exp Hematol 2000;28:1096–1104.

16 Pule M, Savoldo B, Myers GD, Rossig C, et al: Virus-specific T cells engineered to coexpress tumor-specific receptors: persistence and antitumor activity in individuals with neuroblastoma Nat Med 2008;14: 1264–1270.

17 Schulz AS, Glatting G, Hoenig M, Schuetz C, Gatz SA, Grewendorf S, Sparber-Sauer M, Muche R, Blumstein N, Kropshofer G, Suttorp M, Bunjes D, Debatin KM, Reske SN, Friedrich W: Radioimmunotherapy-based conditioning for hematopoietic cell transplantation in children with malignant and nonmalignant diseases. Blood 2011;117:4642–4650.

18 Chiesa R, Veys P: Reduced-intensity conditioning for allogeneic stem cell transplant in primary immune deficiencies. Expert Rev Clin Immunol 2012; 8:255–266.

19 Amrolia P, Gaspar B, Hassan A, et al: Non-myeloablative stem cell transplantation for congenital immunodeficiencies. Blood 2000;96:1239–1246.

20 Rao K, Amrolia PJ, Jones A, et al: Improved survival after unrelated donor bone marrow transplant in children with primary immunodeficiency using a reduced intensity conditioning regimen. Blood 2005; 105:879–885.

21 Cohen JM, Sebire NJ, Harvey J, et al: Successful treatment of lymphoproliferative disease complicating primary immunodeficiency/immunodysregulatory disorders with reduced-intensity allogeneic stem cell transplantation Blood 2007;110:2209–2214.

22 Shenoy S, Grossman WJ, DiPersio J, et al: A novel reduced-intensity stem cell transplant regimen for nonmalignant disorders. Bone Marrow Transplant 2005;35:345–352.

23 Jacobsohn DA, Duerst R, Tse W, et al: Reduced intensity haemopoietic stem-cell transplantation for treatment of non-malignant diseases in children. Lancet 2004;364:156–162.

24 Dennison D, Al Zadjali S, Tauro M, et al: Reduced-intensity conditioning with single daily dose intravenous busulfan, fludarabine and ATG for patients with primary immunodeficiency. Abstract 34th Annual Meeting of the European Group for Blood and Marrow Transplantation, Florence, 2008.
25 Horn B, Baxter-Lowe LA, Englert L, et al: Reduced intensity conditioning using intravenous busulfan, fludarabine and rabbit ATG for children with non-malignant disorders and CML. Bone Marrow Transplant 2006;37:263–269.
26 Güngör T, Albert M, Schanz U, Slatter M, et al: Low-dose busulfan/full-dose fludarabine-based reduced-intensity conditioning in 30 high-risk paediatric and adult chronic granulomatous disease patients. Abstract 37th Annual Meeting of the European Group for Blood and Marrow Transplantation, Florence, 2008.
27 Casper J, Knauf W, Blau I, et al: Treosulfan/fludarabine: a new conditioning regimen in allogeneic transplantation. Ann Hematol 2004;83(suppl 1): S70–S71.
28 Slatter MA, Rao K, Amrolia P, Flood T, Abinun M, Hambleton S, Nademi Z, Goulden N, Davies G, Qasim W, Gaspar HB, Cant A, Gennery AR, Veys P: Treosulfan-based conditioning regimens for hematopoietic stem cell transplantation in children with primary immunodeficiency: United Kingdom experience. Blood 2011;117:4367–4375.
29 Burroughs LM, Storb R, Leisenring WM, et al: Intensive postgrafting immune suppression combined with nonmyeloablative conditioning for transplantation of HLA-identical hematopoietic cell grafts: results of a pilot study for treatment of primary immunodeficiency disorders. Bone Marrow Transplant 2007;40:633–642.
30 Straathof KC, Rao K, Eyrich M, et al: Haemopoietic stem cell transplantation with antibody-based minimal intensity conditioning regimen for children with severe organ toxicity or DNA repair disorders. Lancet 2009;374:912–920.
31 Bradley MB, Satwani P, Baldinger L, et al: Reduced intensity allogeneic umbilical cord blood transplantation in children and adolescent recipients with malignant and non-malignant diseases. Bone Marrow Transplant 2007;40:621–631.
32 Morio T, Atzuta I, et al: Outcome of unrelated umbilical cord blood transplantation in 88 patients with primary immunodeficiency in Japan. Br J Haematol 2011;154:363–372.
33 Horwitz ME, Barrett AJ, Brown MR, et al: Treatment of chronic granulomatous disease with nonmyeloablative conditioning and a T-cell-depleted hematopoietic allograft. N Engl J Med 2001;344:881–888.
34 Ozsahin H, Cavazzana-Calvo M, Notarangelo LD, et al: Long-term outcome following hematopoietic stem cell transplantation in Wiskott-Aldrich syndrome: collaborative study of the European Society for Immunodeficiencies and the European Group for Blood and Marrow Transplantation. Blood 2008; 111:439–445.
35 Pai SY, DeMartiis D, Forino C, et al: Stem cell transplantation for the Wiskott-Aldrich syndrome: a single-center experience confirms efficacy of matched unrelated donor transplantation. Bone Marrow Transplant 2006;38:671–679.
36 Marsh RA, Vaughn G, Kim AH, et al: Reduced-intensity conditioning significantly improves survival of patients with hemophagocytic lymphohistiocytosis undergoing allogeneic hematopoietic cell transplantation. Blood 2010;116:5824–5831.
37 Qasim W, Cavazzana-Calvo M, Davies EG, et al: Allogeneic hematopoietic stem-cell transplantation for leukocyte adhesion deficiency. Pediatrics 2009;123: 836–840.
38 Iannone R, et al: Results of minimally toxic nonmyeloablative transplantation in patients with sickle cell anemia and beta-thalassemia. Biol Blood Marrow Transplant 2003;9:519–528.
39 Bernardo ME, Piras E, Vacca A, Giorgiani G, Zecca M, Bertaina A, Pagliara D, Contoli B, Pinto RM, Caocci G, Mastronuzzi A, La Nasa G, Locatelli F: Allogeneic hematopoietic stem cell transplantation in thalassemia major: results of a reduced-toxicity conditioning regimen based on the use of treosulfan. Blood 2012;120:473–476.

Dr. Paul Veys, BMT Director
Great Ormond Street Hospital
Great Ormond Street
London WC1N 3JH (UK)
E-Mail paul.veys@gosh.nhs.uk

Thomas AE, Halsey C (eds): Controversies in Pediatric and Adolescent Hematology.
Pediatr Adolesc Med. Basel, Karger, 2014, vol 17, pp 135–150 (DOI: 10.1159/000350351)

Can Iron Chelators Replace Stem Cell Transplantation in the Treatment of Thalassaemia Syndromes?

Phil J. Darbyshire

Birmingham Children's Hospital, Birmingham, UK

Abstract

This article looks back on the development of both stem cell transplantation and iron chelation in the treatment of thalassaemia major. The parallel evolution of these two alternative treatments in the 1980s and 1990s, without the benefit of an appropriate clinical trial, has left us assessing the long-term use of desferrioxamine and transplant from matched family donors largely from single-centre studies. This has made genuine comparison much more difficult. It is clear that both treatment options can produce good long-term outcomes. We have now seen that the use of combination therapy with deferiprone and desferrioxamine produces major benefits in reduction in death from cardiac iron overload; more recently, the newer oral chelation agent deferasirox has emerged as a significant advance, and it is expected that the improvements in control of iron overload seen with this agent will be translated into major benefits for patients. The last 10 years have seen alternative donor transplants being evaluated in thalassaemia, this includes both the use of matched adult volunteer donors, related and unrelated cords as well as haploidentical grafts. There are good results published using all these donor types, certainly sufficiently good to be now considered as therapeutic options, the latter probably for higher risk patients. The decision-making process around treatment options in patients with thalassaemia is complex, involving family preferences, financial options as well as the purely medical decisions based on donor availability and medical progress on iron chelating drugs. Advances in both transplantation and chelation have significantly broadened the options available. Discussion about these options must be led by experienced teams, the dialogue should not be directive or undertaken under any time pressure, and it must always retain the best interest of the affected child as the paramount consideration.

Copyright © 2014 S. Karger AG, Basel

Stem cell transplant (SCT) offers at present the only curative option in the treatment of transfusion-dependent thalassaemia major (TM). Whilst the procedure is in many ways similar to SCT for malignant conditions, there are some important differences in both the technology employed, the distribution of complications seen and crucially, the fact that in most instances quality of life decisions are perhaps more central to the decision to graft, there being usually a medical alternative available to SCT.

It could be argued that the most important complication of SCT, that of graft-versus-host (GVH) disease, is occasionally of some value in malignant disease, in terms of reduction in relapse risk via a graft-versus-leukaemia effect; such arguments do not apply in non-malignant disorders and, in SCT for TM in particular, bad GVH is an outcome to be avoided if at all possible.

There have been important advances in SCT for TM in recent years which must be considered alongside advances in iron chelation therapy. The article attempts to ask and hopefully discuss the question of whether these changes have altered the way we should approach treatment recommendations in TM.

This subject will be approached by first of all looking at the history of chelation and stem cell transplantation separately in the treatment of TM. It will then look at the current situation and the future. Discussion will be confined to transfusion-dependent TM that either is using chelation therapy or would need to do so. It is not going to delve into the intricacies of thalassaemia intermedia syndromes, although the discussion about risk benefit of SCT versus medical treatments may still apply.

The term SCT will be used throughout the article to refer to all types of graft, but different donor sources will be referred to where relevant.

One of the challenges in writing an article such as this is in attempting to objectively assess what future developments in both chelation and SCT may bring in the next decade as they may conceivably have to be brought into consideration in treatment decisions. Despite significant advances in both treatment modalities, there remain significant gaps in our knowledge around the very long-term outcomes of both SCT and chelation.

It is worth noting at the beginning that this article is written from the point of view of therapy in the developed world. Later discussion will focus on how different the risk benefit analysis may be when considering treatment in less developed countries or indeed, decisions taken by individuals returning from developed to less developed countries.

Historic Perspective

In assessing and comparing the role of any therapy in TM, it is important to look at the alternative treatment options available at the time. Ideally, this should have been assessed by a randomised controlled study, comparing SCT against the best available chelation treatment. Such studies are notoriously difficult to undertake in SCT. There are major difficulties around consent, as well as in many instances, significant patient and physician bias; suffice to say, such a study of chelation versus SCT has never taken place. Whilst in retrospect one might look back and consider it a shame such a study never occurred, it is never realistically likely to take place in future years. We are, instead, left to rely largely on outcomes from individual centres, registry studies or larger multi-centre studies in the case of chelation therapy. In recent years, there have been some randomised studies in chelation, particularly around the development of deferasirox. The author is aware of none involving randomisation to SCT or medical therapy in the setting of TM.

It is worth reviewing the pathology of iron overload before assessing what was the state of the art in chelation treatment at the time of the first SCTs in the 1980s, and how therapy was beginning to modify the natural history of transfusional iron overload.

It is recognised that the heart, liver, pancreas, anterior pituitary, thyroid and parathyroid glands are the key organs affected by iron deposition. The damage to these organs is mediated by free radical generation by unbound iron. This causes both fibrosis and cell death. The pattern of iron deposition is now well established, with accumulation initially in macrophages of the liver, spleen and bone marrow and, later, when these storage sites are overwhelmed, deposition spreads to hepatocytes and then to endocrine tissues. Finally, deposition begins to occur in the heart. Different organs display different sensitivity to iron damage. It is now clear that the endocrine system is the most sensitive, with pubertal failure continuing to be seen in adequately chelated individuals. This pattern of deposition is responsible for the clinical features of transfusional iron overload; liver fibrosis with eventual cirrhosis, growth and pubertal failure and, finally, heart failure. Before the introduction of modern chelation therapy, heart failure was the cause of death in the majority of patients with transfusional iron overload, typically occurring in teenage or early adult life.

Pre-eminent amongst the early reports of SCT [1–3] are those of the Italian group headed originally by Professor Lucarelli from Pesaro. This group published a series of papers, starting in the 1980s and continuing until the 1990s. The group initially mainly confined SCT to the use of matched family donors. During that period, over 1,000 unselected TM patients were transplanted in Pesaro, with an overall 20 years thalassaemia-free survival of 73%, all of whom received transplants from an HLA-identical family member.

Chelation Therapy

At the time of the initial reports of SCT, regular blood transfusion and chelation with desferrioxamine (DFO) was the standard treatment in clinical practice [4, 5]. Chelation had only been in use in significant numbers of patients for around 10 years and it was really not clear at that time that all the clinical features associated with transfusional overload would be prevented by maintaining a negative iron balance. Whilst there was the hope that such therapy would be effective in the long term, the data were not yet sufficiently mature to be certain. Data on the effect of DFO on cardiac function began to appear in the mid-1980s [6]. It was, however, already clear that long-term medical therapy with transfusion and parenteral DFO was very onerous, maintaining compliance was difficult and such therapy was very expensive. In addition, in many countries, there was a significant risk at the time of hepatitis C transmission. This was the background in which SCT for TM was evolving in the 1980s. We now know that effective chelation therapy has reduced the cardiac mortality of TM to less than 1% in recent cohorts of patients [7].

Chelation therapy has improved greatly from the era of injectable DFO. The major advance that seems to have been mainly responsible for the decline in cardiac deaths was the addition of oral deferiprone to injectable DFO, so-called combination treatment [8, 9]. Deferiprone has only recently being licensed in the US and Canada and there is no doubt that the use of the drug has dramatically reduced cardiac deaths, as well as significantly improving the quality of life for many patients, by reducing reliance on injectable DFO. The major concern with deferiprone remains its unpredictable propensity to cause severe neutropenia [10, 11]. It is a drug that remains useful, particularly in patients with cardiac iron deposition, it does, however, require close monitoring.

More recently, an alternative chelating drug, deferasirox, has been shown to be an effective agent in randomised clinical trials and has been licensed [12, 13]. Experience with this once daily oral agent in both TM and sickle cell disease is now extensive. It is effective and, as long as properly monitored, has a reasonable safely margin [14]. Reversible effects on both renal and liver function are seen and it does not cause neutropenia. Our experience with this drug in Birmingham in over 100 transfusion-dependent children suggests that over 80% will tolerate the drug long term; gastrointestinal side effects, including very rarely gastrointestinal bleeding, being the main reasons for failure. Despite the drug dramatically improving the quality of life for these children and families compared to life using a DFO infuser 5–6 nights weekly for 12 h each night, compliance remains a major problem, many families needing continued support from medical, nursing and psychology staff to maintain a negative iron balance.

This section would not be complete without mention of the role of MRI techniques [15, 16] in the evaluation of cardiac and liver iron deposition. These techniques (T2* MRI for cardiac evaluation and, more recently, FerriScan to assess hepatic iron) have now been well correlated against tissue liver iron concentration and cardiac ejection fraction. They provide a quick accurate quantitative assessment of tissue iron that can be readily repeated to document the impact of chelation therapy. This provides both patients and medical staff with the data needed to tailor or individualise chelation therapy based on drug history and tolerability, patient preferences and the degree of deposition in different organs.

Despite these excellent results, complications are not infrequent. In one Italian study evaluating long-term DFO use [7], hypogonadism was the most frequent complication, affecting 54% of the patients, followed by hypothyroidism (11%) and diabetes (6%). In addition, with increasing age of the patients, new life-threatening complications are being recognised, including severe thrombo-embolic events, pulmonary hypertension, hepatocellular carcinoma and pseudoxanthoma elasticum.

There is now a much wider range of chelation options available and if a negative iron balance is maintained from an early age, there is a good prospect of not only freedom from liver and cardiac disease but also better growth and fertility.

Stem Cell Transplant

It is worth also remembering the environment within which these first SCTs took place. SCT, even from matched family donors, was a hazardous procedure and to see reports of transplant-related mortality of 15–20% was not unusual. This was balanced by the fact that TM was still seen as a disorder carrying a high risk of death from cardiac disease.

The original results, from Lucarelli and the Pesaro group, were excellent, with an initial overall survival of 77% in a large group of patients. They developed a prognostic index to predict transplant outcome in patients younger than age 17 [3]. In essence, there were three criteria all related to iron burden: (1) quality of chelation received before transplantation, (2) hepatomegaly, and (3) the presence of liver fibrosis at a pre-transplant liver biopsy. These variables divided patients into three groups based on having none, one/two, or all three of the risk factors. Overall, survival and thalassaemia-free survival were significantly different in the three groups: 94 and 87% in the low-risk group, 84 and 81% in the intermediate-risk group, and 70 and 58% in the high-risk group, respectively.

Chronic GVH disease proved rare, being seen at grade three or four in 2–5% of children. The results of matched family grafts in adult patients were not as good as those achieved in children, with overall and thalassaemia-free survivals of 65 and 62%, respectively, and a transplant-related mortality rate of 35%, infections being the most common cause of death [17]. The precise reasons why graft rejection is seen more commonly following grafting for TM than other conditions remains unclear. It is likely that repeated exposure to blood products, expanded bone marrow mass and the fact that patients undergoing SCT for TM have not been exposed to prior chemotherapy, with its effect upon the immune system, all contribute.

The paradox at the time was that the group that did best with transplant were precisely the group who were doing best with chelation treatment. Conversely, the poorly compliant patients with higher iron loads and adults who really need SCT did less well [18]. This paradox remains to some extent the same today, despite major improvement in SCT outcomes in recent years for this higher risk group.

There was at the time, some considerable initial debate about the results achieved by the Italian group (mainly from within SCT circles) [19]. The results were significantly better than were being achieved at the time by other groups dealing mainly with patients with malignant disease; the reason for this being probably the age of the children when grafted combined, with the fact they were usually free of the toxicities and infection so often seen in children with malignant disease coming to transplant. Subsequently, other groups confirmed the excellent results being seen from Italy [20]. Measured against these initially excellent results were the inevitable consequences of the alkylating agents used in the conditioning therapy leading to infertility in both males and females [21], although rare spontaneous pregnancies have been reported. It is worth noting again that hypogonadism and problems with fertility are also common in medically treated patients [7].

There have been relatively few series reporting long-term follow-up of a group of survivors' post-SCT [22, 23]. It is clear that those children transplanted late with high iron levels will continue to be at risk of endocrine dysfunction, particularly pubertal failure. In general, however, long-term outcomes are excellent; with very small risks of late graft rejection or second malignancy.

Publications documenting quality of life are similarly relatively few [24]. Those that do exist, in general show excellent outcomes for those unaffected by GVH. The author has seen several families where failure to pass on information about infertility at an appropriate age has caused significant and preventable psychological morbidity. It is important not to lose contact with the post-SCT survivor. There may be issues of fertility and genetic risk that require intervention many years post-graft. It quickly became apparent that the benefits of SCT are maximal in a young child transplanted before the child was exposed to the cumulative effects of high levels of iron over many years. The cumulative damage of years of exposure to high iron levels is not reversible by SCT. Also apparent was the need to rapidly reduce the iron burden post graft [25]. It is our practice to use continuous low dose intravenous DFO during transplant and begin iron removal, with a venesection programme, at around 6 months post-transplant, until normal iron stores are documented; this option being safer and cheaper than using drug-based iron removal regimen.

In summary, the use of SCT evolved at a time when TM was just emerging from an era of being an essentially fatal disorder. Growth and pubertal failure remained common, despite the use of increasingly effective chelation regimes. These regimes required parenteral administration of DFO and were onerous for children, affected adults and their supporting families. Death from cardiac disease was still being regularly seen.

In this setting, SCT from matched family members was an attractive life-saving option. Most who had a matched donor proceeded with the transplant. Does it remain such an attractive option in the era of effective oral chelation, where for many the quality of life may now be rather better?

The Current Situation

The excellent results achieved from Italy have been reproduced by other groups in the UK and Europe. There have been significant advances in the conditioning schedules used in higher risk patients [18]. The use of hydroxycarbamide pre-graft and the use of less toxic conditioning regimes have allowed successful grafts to be undertaken in higher risk patients, bringing results close to the levels seen in class 1 low-risk patients. Despite improvements many clinicians remain wary of undertaking grafts in these higher risk patients. It would certainly be advisable to attempt to reduce the risk with intensive chelation prior to grafting. We now quote a TRM of less than 5% in discussion with families when considering a SCT from a matched family member, with a similar rejection risk. There have been attempts to modify conditioning regimes [26], but none has provided significantly superior results to using a backbone of busulphan and cyclophosphamide within conditioning regimes. One recent publication which shows equivalent results between matched family donors and unrelated donors does postulate treosulphan as a superior condition agent. it is difficult to assess the true value of treosulphan but there is good reason to believe it may be less toxic as a conditioning agent, certainly the DFS and OS of 84 and 93%, respectively, in a group of 40 patients transplanted from unrelated donors is impressive [27].

It has been unusual in the UK to offer grafts from volunteer unrelated donors (VUD). The reason for this has been 2-fold. Firstly, the great majority of patients with TM are from the South Asian Pakistani community where first cousin marriage is still a common practice. This tends to increase the chances of finding a matched family member as a donor source. It is often worth looking for a matched donor within the extended family in these circumstances. Unfortunately, to identify a molecularly matched VUD from the still predominantly Caucasian donor panels is rare. The second factor has been the perception that GVH remains slightly more common in VUD grafts. Recent evidence suggests this may not now be correct. A multi-centre GITMO (Gruppo Italiano Trapianto Midollo Osseo) study, reported results from 68 TM patients, all transplanted from a matched unrelated donor [28]. The age range of this group of paediatric and adult patients was from 2 to 37 years, with a median age of 15 years. Overall, survival and thalassemia-free survival were 79 and 66%, respectively. In the group of 30 paediatric patients in the two lower risk categories, overall survival and thalassemia-free survival were 97 and 80%. In the high-risk group, however, outcomes were less favourable at 65 and 54%. Other reports in recent years have shown good results using well-matched VUD. Most recently, a group from China [29] have published some very encouraging results. They used a transplant protocol based on intravenous busulphan, cyclophosphamide, fludarabine, and thiotepa, in 52 patients using allogeneic peripheral blood stem cell transplantation (PBSCT) from unrelated donors (UD) with well-matched human leukocyte antigens. The median age at transplantation was 6.0 years (range 0.6–15.0). The estimated 3-year overall survival and TM-free survival were 92.3% and 90.4% in the UD-PBSCT group. The cumulative incidences of graft rejection and grade III–IV acute graft versus host disease were 1.9 and 9.6%, respectively, in the UD-PBSCT group. They found a transplant-related mortality of 7.7% in the UD-PBSCT group and 10.0% in a matched sibling donor SCT group using the same protocol; the latter, perhaps, a little higher than would be expected. These, however, are clearly excellent results and it is now increasingly clear that similar results can be obtained using well-matched volunteer donors, in the setting of TM as continue to be achieved using matched family donors.

In recent years, other alternative donor sources have also been shown to produce excellent results. The initial results using matched family cord donors suggested a higher rejection rate but Eurocord data, published in 2005, showed that equivalent results could be obtained using matched related cord material [30]. The Eurocord study documented thirty three grafts in patients with TM: 20/33 Lucarelli class 1 10/33 class 2; there were no high risk patients. They were, in the main, conditioned in a conventional way with busulphan and cyclophosphamide. ATG or thiotepa was added to the preparatory regime in 26/33 patients.

Overall survival was excellent at 100%, 7/33 patients experienced primary graft failure but were able to be rescued by either re-graft or reinfusion of autologous cells. Event free survival of the class 1 patients was 89%, reducing to 62% in the class 2 patients. The risk of GVH was modest with some 11% getting significant acute GVH and 6% chronic GVH. The median cell dose was 4.0×10^6/l. It was clear that the use of an additional agent reduced the risk of graft rejection. It was also obvious that the use of Methotrexate to prevent GVH was associated with a higher risk of graft rejection.

A large international study retrospectively comparing matched related cord blood to bone marrow recipients (each matched for age, risk, and centre experience) in TM has begun to yield comparable results with less GVH occurrence [31]. In this study, overall survival, thalassaemia-free survival, acute GVH, and chronic GVH were 95, 88, 20 and 12% for bone marrow recipients (n = 389, mean age = 8 years), respectively, and 96, 81, 10 and 5% for cord blood recipients (n = 70, mean age = 6 years), respectively. Almost all patients included belonged to the Pesaro 'good-risk' categories.

There is now increasing recognition that successful cord grafting in TM requires a higher cell dose, as well as the omission of methotrexate from post-GVH prophylaxis. These modifications are currently producing results similar to those seen using bone marrow as a stem cell source. Most would now accept that with careful attention to cell dose and, if necessary, even a small top up bone marrow collection, identical results can be obtained from matched family cords compared to using adult bone marrow donors.

A recent study from Taiwan documents the feasibility of using unrelated cord blood transplantation in TM [32]. Forty transplants were performed in 35 patients between October 2003 and September 2009. HLA matching at enrolment was 6/6 (n = 8), 5/6 (n = 16), 4/6 (n = 27), or 3/6 (n = 1) by low-resolution HLA-A, HLA-B, and high-resolution DRB1. These patients received non-manipulated grafts without ex vivo expansion or T cell depletion. The median number of nucleated and CD34+ cells infused was 7.8×10^7/kg (range $2.8–14.7 \times 10^7$/kg) and 4.0×10^5/kg (range $1.7–19.9 \times 10^5$/kg), respectively. The 5-year overall survival and thalassaemia-free survival after the first transplant were 88.3 and 73.9%, respectively. The cumulative incidence of TRM at 2 years was 11.7%. Fourteen patients developed chronic skin GVHD, 30 patients were alive and transfusion-independent between 6 and 76 months post-transplant (median 36 months). The authors comment that the data compare acceptably with the survival rates of related-donor SCT for TM and suggest that patients without an available HLA-compatible sibling, but who have well-matched unrelated cord donors, should also be considered for cord grafts. Whilst these results are excellent, the overall mortality rate and the risk of chronic GVH are both slightly higher than would be expected in grafts using matched family members and it would perhaps be prudent to await a few more data on the degree of matching required before embarking on large-scale programmes of less well matched 4/6 or 3/6 cord transplants. It should be added perhaps that the study quoted above is giving the best results to date, others seeing both high rejection and high mortality in the setting of unrelated cord grafts.

The use of unrelated cord material is a potentially attractive option, particularly for individuals from minority communities, given the less stringent matching that is acceptable when using this donor source. Such a donor source would significantly expand the number of children being able to be offered grafts. It seems likely that if a good match (6/6 or 5/6) can be found with a high cell dose, then this would seem to be an acceptable option.

Attempts have been made at utilising reduced intensity grafting. Again, the numbers of such procedures undertaken has, to date, been small [33]. At present, the results, perhaps not surprisingly, show a rejection rate that is too high for routine use. A better understanding of the problem of mixed chimerism post-graft, combined with post-graft interventions to favour the engrafted cells, are needed before reduced intensity procedures succeed in TM. There is no doubt that such a regime, if available, would quickly find favour; the risk of infertility being, at present, a significant barrier impacting on the decision of families not to proceed with SCT.

Haploidentical related donors after positive selection of $CD34^{+}$ cells have been used in a small series of 22 TM patients [34, 35]. In this series, there were 2 deaths, 6 recurrences of thalassemia, and 14 patients with sustained engraftment. The recent low TRM seen using haploidentical grafts by the Sodani group is encouraging and this type of graft should now be more widely and carefully evaluated in some high-risk patients.

The present situation, in terms of SCT, can be summed up by saying that excellent results continue to be the norm using matched family donors, with matched cord donors with adequate cell dose producing similar results. The results of grafts from full molecularly matched volunteer donors now in this setting are excellent and, as in malignant disease, are producing similar results to those seen in matched family grafts in well-matched donor/recipient pairs.

Outcomes following well-matched unrelated cord grafts and probably haploidentical grafts are now improving towards those seen in matched family grafts. The situation in both arenas here still needs more information. It seems likely for example that well-matched cords (5/6 or 6/6 with high cell dose) will produce excellent results, lower cell doses and increasing degrees of mismatch doing less well.

The data relating to mismatched volunteer donors, and reduced intensity grafts do not yet produce results sufficiently good to recommend them for a child coping well with chelation. There are, however, children who may have specific complications or drug intolerance in which such procedures may offer a real chance of cure.

We now have more mature data on the long-term use of chelating agents, but do not yet have mature data relating to the impact of deferasirox on growth and endocrine function. The essential message remains that virtually the only factor which determines long-term survival is the ability to tolerate chelation long-term with either desferrioxamine or a combination of deferiprone and desferrioxamine. Many studies now document the importance of maintaining a negative iron balance, those unable to do so showing higher rates of organ dysfunction and premature death usually from cardiac disease.

There does, however, continue to be significant endocrine dysfunction even in patients who have been reasonably well chelated. In 2006, De Sanctis et al. [36] found that of a group of 238 children receiving long-term desferrioxamine therapy, 26 patients (12.4%) had growth hormone insufficiency, 5 patients (2.1%) had primary hypothyroidism and 4 patients (1.7%) had hypoparathyroidism. Delayed puberty was present in 18.4% of boys and 17.7% of girls.

We have seen modern chelation therapy transform the outlook of TM, with dramatic reductions in death from cardiac disease particularly being seen in recent years. Despite this, there remains for these adult patients, a significant burden of chronic disease, the need to maintain a regular blood transfusion programme, the risk of fractures related to osteoporosis in adult life, the risk of diabetes mellitus and, often, difficulties with fertility. There is also a real long-term social and psychological impact in living with a chronic disorder, which is harder to quantify with many families and patients wanting to be free of the long-term dependence upon medicine.

There is no doubt that the potential 'game changer' may be the new oral chelator deferasirox. This drug has been licensed for use now for over 6 years. It was subject to rigorous clinical trials within randomised studies, being compared with DFO. In essence, it is a drug that will usually produce negative iron balance at a dose of 30 mg/kg/day. Recent data suggest the dose can be escalated to 40 mg/kg/day, if needed. The most troubling toxicities for the patients are gastrointestinal disturbance with abdominal discomfort, diarrhoea and vomiting. Gastrointestinal bleeding has also been recorded and is warned of in the drug's summary of product characteristics. A dose-dependent increase in creatinine occurs in about a third of patients which, in the majority, resolves without dose adjustment. In our experience of a clinic of around 100 children on this agent, we have managed to successfully establish around 80% of children on the drug with failure usually being due to persistent GI disturbance. The drug needs to be taken once daily as a rather gritty and not particularly pleasant suspension. Despite being a once daily oral medication, long-term compliance remains a significant issue, many children requiring long-term support to achieve this. There is now increasing evidence showing the impact of the drug on maintaining a negative iron balance and its impact on keeping both liver and cardiac iron levels low (as assessed by MRI techniques). As yet, long-term data on the impact of tighter control of iron levels on growth and pubertal development is scanty.

The hope is that the endocrine system, the organ most sensitive to high iron levels, will be protected by better control of iron load over a prolonged time period.

There are isolated case reports of renal impairment, mostly in patients with sickle cell disease, but there does not seem, at present, to be a significant risk of permanent renal impairment. However, continued long-term surveillance is essential, to ensure there are no unexpected late effects of this agent.

In essence, we now have, in deferasirox, a once daily oral medication which will maintain body iron stores at modest levels in most people with TM. In our centre, we have a cohort of teenagers using this agent with no evidence of excess iron deposition in heart or liver. They are growing and passing through puberty quite normally. Whilst there are still unanswered questions about any very long-term toxicity of the drug, with as yet modest data on growth and development in children on the drug, what data we have suggest the drug will certainly keep them free of cardiac and liver iron toxicity and, if started early, we hope will produce a much improved pattern of growth and development in the cohort as a whole. Admittedly, this remains in a setting of maintaining usually a 3- to 4-weekly long-term transfusion programme.

Socio-Economic Considerations

One cannot discuss treatment options in thalassaemia or, indeed, sickle cell disease without mention of socio-economic factors. A very large majority of patients with TM live today in non-industrialised countries, in which availability of these effective therapies is improving, but is still very limited. A recent paper indicated that more than 330,000 haemoglobinopathy-affected infants are born annually (83% sickle cell disorders, 17% thalassaemias) and the large majority of these patients are born and live in the developing world [37]. The UK, in contrast, has around 40 new births per year with TM. Hence, the great majority of TM exists in less developed healthcare systems. It is estimated that the majority remains either untreated or minimally treated and most of these children die during childhood. Countries with less developed health services have responded in different ways to the challenge of TM. Probably the most logical and, ultimately, the most cost effective health interventions are population-based education and screening programmes aimed at offering the option of pre-natal diagnosis, with the expectation, in many instances, of selective termination of affected children.

Once these children with TM begin treatment with transfusion (either intermittent or regular), they begin to live beyond childhood and will be at risk of the long-term problems of iron overload. TM is expensive to treat long-term using conventional transfusion and chelation.

One also has to factor in the costs of monitoring therapy with MRI techniques, as well as coping with complications such as heart disease and diabetes. The precise costs obviously vary between different countries, but in the UK, an annual cost for conventional transfusion and chelation is estimated at around GBP 30,000 per year, increasing with age as iron-related complications occur.

The cost of SCT varies widely between different countries and health care systems, but in the UK currently, a figure of GBP 100,000 for a SCT from a matched donor in a young child would be not far short of the mark. Leaving aside the precise figures, which are subject to very wide variation from country to country and between different health care models, there is no doubt that the lifetime cost of an effective modern transfusion and chelation programme far exceeds the one-off cost of SCT, assuming the transplant is undertaken at a sufficiently early age to prevent long-term problems associated with iron overload. What data we have suggest, apart from the small number with chronic GVH, that the burden of long-term disability in SCT survivors is modest, certainly not high enough to counter-balance the financial advantage of SCT.

It is quite clear, for a country with limited health resources, that SCT, particularly from a matched family member, is an attractive therapeutic option. Despite the excellent results now being seen using alternative donor sources, the high procurement costs, particularly of cord material, will remain a barrier in some countries. Hence, it is really only in well-developed insurance-based or state-funded health care systems that there is a genuine choice in terms of using SCT or medical therapy, the lifetime costs of effective transfusion and chelation being essentially beyond the means of most individuals living in health care systems who do not have insurance-based or state support. These considerations do alter, significantly, the health care decisions of families and patients who are returning to live in less well-developed countries; such individuals often accepting much higher levels of risk in terms of transplant outcome than we would expect in an indigenous UK family.

The Future

How should one now approach a child with transfusion-dependent TM? SCT remains the only curative option available at present, and the availability of oral chelators has not altered this position. We do, however, now have a much clearer position about the risks and benefits of different approaches, as well as socio-economic considerations.

Are there new treatment modalities arriving that are likely to influence this discussion? I have been awaiting the arrival of gene therapy for haemoglobin disorders for over 20 years now. Whilst there has been progress, the clinical use in TM remains some years in the future. A more immediate prospect may be a better (more palatable and more efficient, with fewer side effects) chelating drug. A report this year on FBS0701 [38] is promising, but seems unlikely to greatly modify this discussion in the next few years.

No prospective randomised clinical trials are now likely to provide a definitive answer to the challenge of choosing between transplant and medical therapy for each individual patient. In the absence of definitive evidence, the decision process is highly individualised and patient-specific. It must consider many factors: age, clinical status, willingness to undergo a toxic treatment, donor match and availability, financial position, compliance with chelation, the ability to adhere to the appropriate transfusion regimes, perceived quality of life, social, family and religious beliefs, family, and other resources available.

Parents of paediatric patients must, of course, take this decision on behalf of the child, at an age when the child themselves will have little or no real input or understanding of the decision taking place.

There is no doubt that the results of SCT, using matched family donors, in young patients with TM are excellent, with most centres now achieving over 90% survival and 85% disease-free survival. This curative option remains an attractive one for many families, despite its well-documented risks.

We would now also recommend undertaking a volunteer donor search for all families without a matched family donor, although, to date, we have not identified a fully matched adult donor in any of our predominantly South Asian children. We would, however, view any such fully matched donor now as equivalent to a matched family donor.

We also undertake a volunteer cord search and would increasingly view a 6/6 or 5/6 high cell dose cord as a donor source, accepting that data not perhaps quite as clear as that for volunteer donors.

The use of haploidentical donors has been undertaken in TM, with some encouraging results. Such procedures do have a place, but need careful discussion based on individual circumstances. The relative merits of a well matched unrelated cord or haploidentical grafts are difficult to balance at present, the former producing a higher TRM, the latter a higher rejection rate, both should only be undertaken by experienced units and outcome data carefully monitored. They are difficult to justify for a child within a supportive family who is maintaining a negative iron balance. Our view has been not to undertake such procedures under these circumstances, preferring increasingly to direct the family towards newer techniques, such as pre-implantation diagnosis, that might allow the possibility of a matched graft. Conversely, for a child struggling to maintain a chelation regime or who has had adverse reactions to chelation drugs, the exploration of alternative donor sources is a valid option given recent encouraging data in TM, we should now be embracing such options as quickly as possible to get the best possible outcomes.

Families take very different views about SCT versus chelation, sometimes very different from their medical attendants with some not wishing to take the small risk of death during the procedure and wishing to preserve fertility while others wishing to press on with SCT at almost any price. Our approach in Birmingham remains to try and discuss SCT in a balanced and open way with all families, under most circumstances offering this as a treatment option, rather than a recommendation. We try to encourage most families considering SCT to embark upon chelation therapy (usually deferasirox) and to get a feel for how life unfolds on long-term transfusion and chelation, giving the positive message that the child should be treated as any other child, at home and at school. The majority of families do still opt to embark on SCT if a family donor is found, but significant proportions choose to remain on medical treatment. It is always difficult to separate out the views of those looking after the families. In general, we do our best not to be directive, as for a child managing a negative iron balance without problems; continued medical therapy is a very reasonable choice. There are circumstances in which a stronger case can be made for SCT; the most common of these in our unit being in families where, for whatever reason, chelation treatment is proving hard to establish or maintain.

There is ample evidence that poor chelation in early life usually translates into poor long-term outcomes. Even if adequate chelation is established in later childhood or teenage years, the exposure to high iron levels does impact on growth and pubertal development. Such families do need intensive support to comply with the chelation regime and should get an honest discussion of the increased long-term risks. Our approach, in such circumstances, is to recommend SCT to the family after a period of intensive supervised chelation prior to the graft.

We would also view a child returning to a less developed part of the world in a different light. Such children may not have regular access to safe red cell transfusion. They may not have the resources needed to buy chelation drugs on a long-term basis. Again, in these circumstances, SCT is likely to be the best option.

One of the difficult situations is the family who wish to have a transplant, despite there being no suitably matched donor available. The view of the family is clearly important. However, as physicians, there is an obligation to put the best interests of the child first. Very often, the desire for SCT, at any cost, may derive from a limited understanding of the disorder and what can reasonably be achieved with medical treatment. In some instances, the views may be coming from other remote family members who may be very poorly informed. It is often worth trying to discuss, with the parents, and, sometimes, the extended family, the therapeutic options available. Certainly, for a child struggling to maintain a chelation regime or who has had adverse reactions to chelation drugs, the early exploration of alternative donor sources is an increasingly valid option.

Conclusion

It is, not surprisingly, impossible to give a simple answer to the original question posed. SCT continues to have a role in the therapy of TM, although, for young people, maintaining a negative iron balance on oral chelators, there is no longer such a strong case to recommend the transplant option. Conversely, better data on the poor outcomes of those who do not manage to maintain a negative iron loads suggest that we should be more proactive in looking at alternative donor options at a young age, in order to optimise outcomes. This discussion around both SCT and medical treatment needs to take place over a prolonged period of time. It should be undertaken in a balanced way by a team with experience of both SCT and medical treatment for TM and must take a wide variety of factors into account. At the heart of any discussion must be the best interest of the child themselves. The most encouraging aspect being that we do now have more treatment options available, both medical and SCT, that represent good long-term therapeutic options. We do, however, need to systematically collect very long-term outcome data to inform discussion in future years.

References

1 Lucarelli G, Polchi P, Izzi T, et al: Allogeneic marrow transplantation for thalassemia. Exp Hematol 1984; 12:676–681.

2 Lucarelli G, Polchi P, Galimberti M, et al: Marrow transplantation for thalassaemia following busulphan and cyclophosphamide. Lancet 1985;i:1355–1357.

3 Lucarelli G, Galimberti M, Polchi P, et al: Bone marrow transplantation in patients with thalassemia. N Engl J Med 1990;322:417–421.

4 Olivieri NF, Nathan DG, MacMillan JH, et al: Survival in medically treated patients with homozygous beta-thalassemia. N Engl J Med 1994;331:574–578.

5 Brittenham GM, Griffith PM, Nienhuis AW, et al: Efficacy of deferoxamine in preventing complications of iron overload in patients with thalassemia major. N Engl J Med 1994;331:567–573.

6 Marcus RE, Davies SC, Bantock HM, Underwood SR, Walton S, Huehns ER: Desferrioxamine to improve cardiac function in iron overloaded patients with thalassaemia major. Lancet 1984;i:392.

7 Borgna-Pignatti C, Rugolotto S, De Stefano P, Zhao H, Cappellini MD, Del Vecchio GC, et al: Survival and complications in patients with thalassemia major treated with transfusion and deferoxamine. Haematologica 2004;89:1187–1193.

8 Pennell DJ, Berdoukas V, Karagiorga M, et al: Randomized controlled trial of deferiprone or deferoxamine in beta-thalassemia major patients with asymptomatic myocardial siderosis. Blood 2006;107: 3738–3744.

9 Tanner MA, Galanello R, Dessi C, et al: A randomized, placebo-controlled, double-blind trial of the effect of combined therapy with deferoxamine and deferiprone on myocardial iron in thalassemia major using cardiovascular magnetic resonance. Circulation 2007;115:1876–1884.

10 Ceci A, Baiardi P, Felisi M, et al: The safety and effectiveness of deferiprone in a large-scale, 3-year study in Italian patients. Br J Haematol 2002;118: 330–336.

11 Cohen AR, Galanello R, Piga A, De Sanctis V, Tricta F: Safety and effectiveness of long-term therapy with the oral iron chelator deferiprone. Blood 2003;102: 1583–1587.

12 Cappellini MD, Cohen A, Piga A, et al: A phase 3 study of deferasirox (ICL670), a once-daily oral iron chelator, in patients with beta-thalassemia. Blood 2006;107:3455–3462.

13 Cappellini MD, Bejaoui M, Agaoglu L, Canatan D, Capra M, Cohen A, Drelichman G, Economou M, Fattoum S, Kattamis A, Kilinc Y, Perrotta S, Piga A, Porter JB, Griffel L, Dong V, Clark J, Aydinok Y: Iron chelation with deferasirox in adult and pediatric patients with thalassemia major: efficacy and safety during 5 years' follow-up. Blood 2011;118:884–893.

14 Cappellini MD, Elalfy MS, Kattamis A, Seymour JF, Lee CL, Porter JB: Efficacy and safety of once-daily, oral iron chelator deferasirox (EXJADE®) in a large group of regularly transfused patients with β-thalassemia major. Blood 2008;112:abstr 3878.

15 Anderson LJ, Westwood MA, Holden S, et al: Myocardial iron clearance during reversal of siderotic cardiomyopathy with intravenous desferrioxamine: a prospective study using T2* cardiovascular magnetic resonance. Br J Haematol 2004;127:348–355.

16 St Pierre TG, Clark PR, Chua-anusorn W, et al: Non-invasive measurement and imaging of liver iron concentrations using proton magnetic resonance. Blood 2005;105:855–861.

17 Lucarelli G, Clift RA, Galimberti M, et al: Bone marrow transplantation in adult thalassemic patients. Blood 1999;93:1164–1167.

18 Lucarelli G, Clift RA, Galimberti M, et al: Marrow transplantation for patients with thalassemia: results in class 3 patients. Blood 1996;87:2082–2088.

19 Lucarelli G, Weatherall DJ: For debate: bone marrow transplantation for severe thalassaemia (1). The view from Pesaro (2). To be or not to be. Br J Haematol 1991;78:300–303.

20 Lawson SE, Roberts IA, Amrolia P, Dokal I, Szydlo R, Darbyshire PJ: Bone marrow transplantation for beta-thalassaemia major: the UK experience in two paediatric centres. Br J Haematol 2003;120:289–295.
21 Vlachopapadopoulou E, Kitra V, Peristeri J, Goussetis E, Karachaliou F, Petropoulos D, Fotinou A, Michalacos S, Graphakos S: Gonadal function of young patients with beta-thalassemia following bone marrow transplantation. J Pediatr Endocrinol Metab 2005;18:477–483.
22 De Sanctis V, Galimberti M, Lucarelli G, Polchi P, Ruggiero L, Vullo C, De Sanctis V, Galimberti M, Lucarelli G, et al: Growth and development in ex-thalassemic patients. Bone Marrow Transplant 1997; 19(suppl 2):126–127.
23 Di Bartolomeo P, Santarone S, Di Bartolomeo E, et al: Long-term results of survival in patients with thalassemia major treated with bone marrow transplantation. Am J Hematol 2008;83:528–530.
24 Clarke SA, Skinner R, Guest J, Darbyshire P, Cooper J, Shah F, Roberts I, Eiser C: Health-related quality of life and financial impact of caring for a child with thalassaemia major in the UK. Child Care Health Dev 2010;36:118–122.
25 Angelucci E, Muretto P, Lucarelli G, et al: Phlebotomy to reduce iron overload in patients cured of thalassemia by bone marrow transplantation. Italian Cooperative Group for Phlebotomy Treatment of Transplanted Thalassemia Patients. Blood 1997;90: 994–998.
26 Bernardo ME, Zecca M, Piras E, et al: Treosulfan-based conditioning regimen for allogeneic haematopoietic stem cell transplantation in patients with thalassaemia major. Br J Haematol 2008;143:548–551.
27 Bernardo ME, Piras E, Vacca A, Giorgiani G, Zecca M, Bertaina A, Pagliara D, Contoli B, Pinto RM, Caocci G, Mastronuzzi A, La Nasa G, Locatelli F: Allogeneic hematopoietic stem cell transplantation in thalassemia major: results of a reduced-toxicity conditioning regimen based on the use of treosulfan. Blood 2012;120:473–476.
28 La Nasa G, Argiolu F, Giardini C, et al: Unrelated bone marrow transplantation for beta-thalassemia patients: the experience of the Italian Bone Marrow Transplant Group. Ann NY Acad Sci 2005;1054: 186–195.
29 Li C, Wu X, Feng X, He Y, Liu H, Pei F, Liao J, He L, Shi L, Li N, Liu Q, Liu S, Chen G, Su Q, Ren Y, Wang Y, Tan W: A novel conditioning regimen improves outcomes in B-thalassemia major patients using unrelated donor peripheral blood stem cell transplantation. Blood 2012;120:3875–3881.
30 Locatelli F, Rocha V, Reed W, et al: Related umbilical cord blood transplantation in patients with thalassemia and sickle cell disease. Blood 2003;101:2137–2143.
31 Kabbara N, Locatelli F, Rocha V, et al: A multicentric comparative analysis of outcomes of HLA identical related cord blood and bone marrow transplantation in patients with beta-thalassemia or sickle cell disease. Biol Blood Marrow Transplant 2008;14:3–4.
32 Jaing T-H, Hung I-J, Yang C-P, Chen S-H, Chung H-T, Tsay P-K, Wen Y-C: Unrelated cord blood transplantation for thalassaemia: a single-institution experience of 35 patients. Bone Marrow Transplant 2012;47:33–39.
33 Bertaina A, Bernardo ME, Mastronuzzi A, La Nasa G, Locatelli F: The role of reduced intensity preparative regimens in patients with thalassemia given hemopoietic transplantation. Ann NY Acad Sci 2010; 1202:141–148.
34 Lucarelli G, Gaziev J: Advances in the allogeneic transplantation for thalassemia. Blood Rev 2008:22: 53–63.
35 Sodani P, Isgro A, Gaziev J, et al: Purified T-depleted, CD34+ peripheral blood and bone marrow cell transplantation from haploidentical mother to child with thalassemia. Blood 2010;115:1296–1302.
36 De Sanctis V, Roos M, Gasser T, Fortini M, Raiola G, Galati MC: Italian Working Group on Endocrine Complications in Non-Endocrine Diseases. J Pediatr Endocrinol Metab 2006;19:471–480.
37 Modell B, Darlison M: Global epidemiology of haemoglobin disorders and derived service indicators. Bull World Health Organ 2008;86:480–487.
38 Neufeld EJ, Galanello R, Viprakasit V, et al: A phase 2 study of the safety, tolerability, and pharmacodynamics of FBS0701, a novel oral iron chelator, in transfusional iron overload. Blood 2012;119:3263–3268.

Dr. Phil J. Darbyshire
Consultant Paediatric Haematologist
Birmingham Children's Hospital
Steelhouse Lane, Birmingham B4 6NH (UK)
E-Mail phil.darbyshire@bch.nhs.uk

Thomas AE, Halsey C (eds): Controversies in Pediatric and Adolescent Hematology.
Pediatr Adolesc Med. Basel, Karger, 2014, vol 17, pp 151–160 (DOI: 10.1159/000350352)

Iron Deficiency: When and Why Oral Iron May Not Be Enough

Shelley E. Crary[a] · George R. Buchanan[b]

[a]Department of Pediatrics, University of Arkansas for Medical Sciences, Little Rock, Ark., and
[b]Department of Pediatrics, University of Texas Southwestern Medical Center, Dallas, Tex., USA

Abstract

Use of intravenous iron in children has been limited due to concerns regarding adverse effects. However, newer preparations of intravenous iron have been shown to be effective and associated with fewer side effects in adults as well as in preliminary studies involving children. Indications for intravenous iron might include iron deficiency secondary to dietary causes, blood loss unresponsive to oral iron and situations where oral iron is ineffective, contraindicated or when functional iron deficiency exists. This review will discuss the various preparations of iron available for parenteral administration and the potential indications for their use in children.

Copyright © 2014 S. Karger AG, Basel

Overview of Iron Deficiency

Prevalence and Etiology

Iron deficiency is the most common mineral deficiency in the world, affecting both high income and developing countries. For example, its prevalence in the United States is highest in toddlers and adolescent females, with rates of 9–14% in both groups [1]. Iron deficiency results from several distinct etiologies with varying prevalence dependent primarily on age. It may be a consequence of inadequate iron endowment at birth. This is usually due to low birth weight and occurs with increased frequency in developing countries where malnutrition is prevalent. Decreased iron intake is most common in infants and young children and results primarily from excessive cow's milk intake, which causes anemia by three primary mechanisms: (1) deficiency of bioavailable iron, (2) microvascular gastrointestinal blood loss when consumed in large quantities, and (3) inhibited duodenal absorption of nonheme iron contained in other foods [2]. Another prevalent etiology for iron deficiency in developed countries is excessive blood loss. This is primarily seen in adolescent, menstruating females but also may occur as a result of recurrent epistaxis or gastrointestinal bleeding accompanying inflammatory bowel disease (IBD) or other anatomic lesions. In low-income tropical countries parasitic infection, most commonly hookworm infestation, is frequently responsible for chronic intestinal bleeding. Rarely, iron deficiency in young patients presents with malabsorption resulting from anatomic, inflammatory or inherited conditions such as defects in the *TMPRSS6* gene. Hereditary hemorrhagic telangiectasia can result in iron deficiency anemia due to recurrent bleeding from mucosal telangiectases or visceral arteriovenous malformations. Iron restricted erythropoiesis or functional iron deficiency, due to disordered iron homeostasis, is yet another indication for iron replacement. This may occur secondary to subacute or chronic inflammatory conditions such as cancer, infections, and autoimmune diseases as well as in patients with chronic renal failure receiving dialysis.

Overview of Iron Absorption

Iron is primarily absorbed from the duodenum in the form of the Fe^{2+} (ferrous) ion or as iron bound to heme. Once either form of iron enters the enterocyte, it is transported by ferroportin across its basolateral membrane and released into the circulation bound by transferrin and carried to sites where the iron will be stored or utilized. The amount of iron absorbed is closely regulated to be equivalent to that which is lost. Iron absorption is increased if iron stores are low (e.g. iron deficiency), with hypoxemia, increased erythropoietic activity, or anemia. Hepcidin is the main regulator of iron absorption. In states of iron deficiency, hypoxia, or anemia, production of hepcidin is downregulated and the transferrin receptor upregulated, thus promoting absorption of iron and utilization of iron stored in macrophages. However, with iron-restricted erythropoiesis, such as occurs with anemia of inflammation, increased production of hepcidin is stimulated by inflammatory cytokines. By subsequently binding to ferroportin it effectively blocks iron absorption from enterocytes and release from macrophages. In addition, erythropoietin production is suppressed relative to the degree of anemia present. Similar mechanisms underlie anemia of chronic renal disease. Erythropoiesis-stimulating agents (ESA) have thus been utilized to treat iron-restricted erythropoiesis, and recent studies have also shown a possible role for parenteral iron replacement in these conditions [3].

Consequences of Iron Deficiency

Iron deficiency is a multisystem disorder which primarily causes anemia and its accompanying clinical sequelae, but cognitive and neurologic deficits are also prevalent. Iron is required for the growth of all cells and plays a particularly important role in the central nervous system, including neuronal and glial metabolism, myelination and production of neurotransmitters [4]. Iron deficiency may cause pica (and accordingly may contribute to increased lead burden), seizures, and, especially when present in children <2 years of age, long-lasting, irreversible neurocognitive and behavioral consequences [5, 6]. Therefore, it is imperative that iron deficiency, if not prevented, is promptly diagnosed and fully treated. The most important strategies for the prevention of iron deficiency in young children are breast feeding (with provision of iron supplements after 5–6 months of age) and avoidance of cow's milk until beyond 1 year of age and subsequent limitation of its intake to less than or equal to 24 ounces (680 ml) daily.

Oral Iron Therapy

Oral iron replacement has been the longstanding treatment of choice for iron deficiency due to inadequate dietary intake or chronic blood loss. Dozens of formulations of oral iron exist but no definitive studies have ever compared the different brands or formulations for efficacy or tolerability. Generally, 3–6 mg/kg/day of elemental iron in divided doses is recommended for successful treatment of moderate-to-severe iron deficiency [7]. This approach is frequently associated with gastrointestinal side effects (such as nausea, constipation and abdominal discomfort), thus limiting adherence to the prescribed treatment course required to treat the anemia and subsequently replete iron stores [8]. In addition, in patients with ongoing blood loss, oral dosing may not provide sufficient iron to overcome the amount that is lost. Patients with malabsorption or functional iron deficiency will also not adequately respond to oral iron. Thus, there are many limitations to the success of oral iron therapy in children of all ages.

Intravenous Iron Therapy

History of Intravenous Iron

The first widely accepted parenteral iron preparation was iron dextran, introduced in the United States in 1954. Until 1992, high-molecular-weight iron dextran (HMWID) (Imferon®, Fisons, UK) was the only parenteral iron formulation available. Due to multiple reports of anaphylactic reactions with this product its use was restricted; many hematologists became apprehensive about the use of intravenous iron in general. Intramuscular Imferon® was in vogue for a while, but the repeated deep buttock injections were painful and the local skin discoloration was problematic. Accordingly, distribution of Imferon was ultimately discontinued in 1992 but was replaced by Dexferrum® (American Regent, Shirley, N.Y., USA), a similar

HMWID preparation, in 1996. Meanwhile, INFeD® (Watson Pharma, Inc., Morristown, N.J., USA), a low-molecular-weight iron dextran (LMWID) associated with far fewer adverse reactions than HMWID was approved for use in the United States in 1991 [9, 10].

As the worldwide requirements for intravenous iron preparations increased, primarily due to the rise in the use of ESA in patients with chronic kidney disease, non-dextran intravenous irons were introduced to the market, including ferric gluconate (Ferrlecit®, Sanofi-Aventis, Paris) in 1999 and iron sucrose (Venofer®, American Regent, Shirley, N.Y., USA) shortly thereafter. These agents have since replaced iron dextran in most dialysis centers due to their perceived improved safety profile [9]. Iron sucrose has also been safely used in children with iron deficiency anemia [11, 12]. A recent study of its use in a diverse group of children without chronic renal failure for whom oral iron was unsuitable or inadequate showed encouraging results [12]. The newest intravenous iron product available on the US market, FDA approved in 2009 and EMA approved in 2012, is ferumoxytol (Feraheme®, Rienso® (EU), AMAG, Lexington, Mass., USA), which was initially designed as a novel imaging contrast agent and has been licensed for the treatment of iron deficiency anemia in adult patients with chronic kidney disease. In Europe, two additional new products have recently been approved, ferric carboxymaltose (Ferinject®, Vifor, Switzerland) and iron isomaltoside 1,000 (Monofer®, Pharmacosmos, Denmark). Both have been heralded as promising improved safety profiles and ease of dosing although currently Ferinject is only licensed for those 14 years and over and Monofer is not licensed for use in children.

Safety of Intravenous Iron Preparations

Most of the available literature comparing the efficacy and safety profiles of various intravenous iron preparations focuses on adults with chronic kidney disease. Although LMWID has a similar but more favorable side effect profile than HMWID which is associated with more serious adverse events, allergic and anaphylactic reactions can occur with both formulations [9, 13] (table 1). For example, direct comparison in 156 adults undergoing dialysis revealed a 3.5% rate of adverse effects with LMWID versus 28.6% with HMWID [14]. Many studies reporting high rates of adverse events with iron dextran do not differentiate between the two forms (HMW vs. LMW), but most reactions were likely related to the former [15]. Almost no clinical trials have yet included children without chronic kidney disease, but two recent studies of children with iron deficiency anemia of various non-renal causes showed that iron sucrose can be safely administered in an outpatient setting with good efficacy [11, 12]. A study of single total dose infusions (rather than repeated dosing) of iron dextran in children with IBD and iron deficiency confirmed its efficacy. Eleven adverse reactions occurred during 119 infusions, but it is unclear whether a LMW or HMW

Table 1. Major adverse drug events of parenteral iron formulations, 2001 through 2003 [9]

Adverse drug events	Ferrlecit (ferrous gluconate) (n = 11,973,800)	Dexferrum (HMWID) (n = 2,563,000)	INFeD (LMWID) (n = 6,690,000)	Venofer (iron sucrose) (n = 8,837,000)	OR dexferrum vs. INFeD (95% CI)	OR ferrlecit vs. INFeD (95% CI)	OR venofer vs. INFeD (95% CI)	OR venofer vs. ferrlecit (95% CI)
Total[a], n (per million)	232 (19.4)	331 (129.2)	269 (40.2)	175 (19.8)	3.2 (2.7–3.8)	0.5 (0.4–0.6)	0.5 (0.4–0.6)	1.0 (0.8–1.2)
Life-threatening[b]	11 (0.9)	29 (11.3)	22 (3.3)	5 (0.6)	3.4 (2.0–5.9)	0.3 (0.1–0.7)	0.2 (0.1–0.4)	0.6 (0.2–1.7)

[a] Includes death, cardiac arrest, coma, anaphylactoid reaction, dyspnea, allergic reaction, abdominal pain, back pain, chest pain, hypotension, nausea, vomiting, and sweating. [b] Includes death, cardiac arrest, coma and anaphylactoid reaction. OR = Odds ratio; n = total number of infusions. Adapted from Chertow et al. [9].

ID was responsible as both formulations were employed in study patients [16]. Total dose infusion of LMW ID has been shown to be effective in a separate study of 31 pediatric patients treated in an outpatient hematology clinic, with minor adverse reactions noted in 9 patients but no anaphylaxis or other serious adverse events [17]. Frequently patients will complain of arthralgia and myalgia during the test dose or subsequent infusion of LMW ID. However, this is generally self-limiting and does not portend more serious reactions, and most patients can successfully receive the complete infusion [18, 19].

The introduction of second-generation intravenous iron formulations, such as iron sucrose and ferric gluconate preparations are effective in the treatment of IDA and are not associated with the serious allergic reactions encountered with intravenous iron dextran. They have favorable safety profiles when compared with the dextran preparations (table 1) but at doses greater than 300 mg patients may experience transient side effects such as hypotension, abdominal pain and nausea/vomiting [20]. These dose-dependent adverse effects are thought to be vasoactive reactions due to circulating free (unbound) iron that occur when transferrin becomes temporarily oversaturated during the infusion. This problem likely results from nondextran iron preparations binding iron less tightly than dextran [20, 21]. Ferumoxytol use in children has been limited, but a preliminary report in 6 children with gastrointestinal disorders supported its safety with doses up to 12 mg/kg (maximum 510 mg, the vial content) given over 15–60 min [22].

Choice of Intravenous Iron Formulation

The selection of intravenous iron preparations will depend on the underlying indication for iron and the clinical setting (table 2). For children with renal failure undergoing dialysis, frequent small doses of a product such as ferric gluconate or iron sucrose would be a good choice given the larger experience with these products and their fa-

Table 2. Comparison of intravenous iron preparations [13]

Generic (trade) name	Currently available intravenous iron preparations						
	iron dextran injection (Dexferrum)	iron dextran injection (INFeD (US); CosmoFer (UK))	sodium ferric gluconate complex (Ferrlecit)	iron sucrose injection (Venofer)	ferumoxytol (Feraheme, Rienso)	iron isomaltoside 1,000 (Monofer)	ferric carboxy-maltose injection (Injectafer (US) Ferinject (EU))
Manufacturer	American Regent Inc.	Watson Pharma-ceuticals Inc.; Pharmacosmos	Sanofi-Aventis Inc.	American regen Inc.	AMAG Pharmaceuticals; Takeda UK Ltd	Pharmacosmos A/S	Luitpold Pharmaceuti-cals; Vifor
Carbohydrate	high-molecular-weight iron dextran	low-molecular-weight iron dextran	gluconate	sucrose	polyglucose sorbitol carboxymethy-lether	oligosaccharide	carboxy-maltose
Molecular weight (Da)	265,000	165,000	289,000–440,000	34,000–60,000	750,000	165,000	150,000
Total dose or >500 mg infusion possible?	yes	yes	no	no	yes	yes	yes
Premedication recommendation	TDI only	TDI only	no	no	no	no	no
Test dose required?	yes	yes	no	no	no	no	no
Iron concentration, mg/ml	50	50	12.5	20	30	100	30
Vial volume, ml	1–2	2	5	5	17	1 and 5 ml^	2 ml
Black box warning	yes	yes	no	no	no	yes^	yes
Preservative	none	none	benzyl alcohol	none	none	none	none
Pediatric FDA approved	yes >4 months	yes >4 months	yes >6 years	no	no	no*	no*
Pediatric EMA approved	no	yes >14 years	no	no	no	no^	yes >14 years

* Not FDA approved for adults. ^ EMA approved >18 years.
TDI = Total dose infusion. Table adapted from Auerbach and Ballard [13].

vorable safety profile. However, in the outpatient pediatric hematology or GI clinic setting it may be preferable to administer a more substantial dose or even total iron deficit correction during a single visit. This approach may improve patient and family adherence and be more cost effective as well. Product choices currently allowing for total dose infusions include low molecular weight iron dextran and ferumoxytol. Although the pediatric data supporting this approach are very limited, the initial reports are encouraging [16, 17, 22].

Patients Who May Benefit from Intravenous Iron

Dietary Iron Deficiency

To our knowledge, there are no comparative studies of intravenous versus oral iron for young children with nutritional iron deficiency anemia. Since side effects of oral iron in 20% or more of patients may limit adherence to prescribed treatment regimens [8, 23], intravenous iron may have a role in rapidly and efficiently correcting iron deficiency in these patients. This strategy may be particularly important in toddlers since iron deficiency can have long-lasting, neurocognitive sequelae. Further study of 'up front' intravenous iron therapy in toddlers with dietary iron deficiency may be warranted, especially with newer intravenous iron agents that potentially allow total dose infusion during a brief, single outpatient visit [24].

Blood Loss

Studies in adults have demonstrated the beneficial results of intravenous iron administration to assure adequate stores that compensate for acute and chronic blood loss. For example, a randomized, controlled trial of intravenous ferric carboxymaltose versus oral ferrous sulfate in women with menorrhagia showed greater rise in hemoglobin concentration and improved quality of life measures when compared to oral iron [25]. Limited data are also available regarding intravenous iron sucrose in children with gastrointestinal blood loss or menorrhagia [12]. It is reasonable to speculate, therefore, that intravenous iron would be more effective and tolerable in children with ongoing blood losses who require high and repetitive doses of oral iron replacement.

Inflammatory Bowel Disease

Evidence supports the efficacy of intravenous rather than oral iron for anemia related to IBD in adults [26], but thus far with limited evidence in children [16]. The 70% prevalence of anemia in children with IBD represents a large population potentially available for comparative effectiveness studies of different intravenous iron preparations.

Functional Iron Deficiency

The most prevalent current indication for intravenous iron in children is chronic kidney disease, especially patients also receiving an ESA. Iron-restricted erythropoiesis due to functional iron deficiency often occurs in this setting, thus limiting ESA effec-

Table 3. Comparison of oral versus intravenous iron treatment

	Oral iron	Intravenous iron
Medication cost	USD 44.00[a]	USD 308.00[b]
Additional financial burden	follow-up clinic visits; loss of work/school	intravenous infusion costs
Adverse effects	moderate to high risk but generally mild, primarily gastrointestinal but may reduce adherence	low risk, but potentially serious
Patient/family burden	potentially great	low
Adherence burdens	daily prolonged therapy	transient discomfort from intravenous infusion
Conventional indications	dietary iron deficiency blood loss	functional iron deficiency, i.e. chronic kidney disease treated with ESA oral iron malabsorption

[a] Based on retail pricing of generic ferrous sulfate 325 mg tablet dosed twice daily for 4 months.
[b] Based on retail pricing of single INFeD 1,000-mg dose.

tiveness. This problem can be overcome by intravenous but not oral iron therapy [3]. All intravenous iron formulations currently available in the US and EU have an FDA or EMA indication for adult patients with chronic kidney disease. Yet only Ferrlicet® and INFeD® have thus far been approved for use in children.

Another setting in which functional iron deficiency occurs is anemia of inflammation. Increasing evidence supports that some affected patients may respond to intravenous iron therapy with or without ESA [27]. This has been most often studied, with varied results, in adults with cancer- or chemotherapy-induced anemia [28, 29]. There have been to date no pediatric studies of intravenous iron in cancer-induced anemia and only one publication on the anemia of inflammation [30]. This is therefore a compelling area for further research.

Conclusions

Intravenous iron has come a long way during the past 50 years. Newer preparations are much safer than the first high-molecular-weight iron dextran products introduced to the market in the 1950s. Despite these advances in safety, the clinical use of intravenous iron outside the chronic kidney disease setting has been limited, in great part due to provider anxiety and misconceptions regarding its safety. Since the efficacy of intravenous iron is undisputed, it should more often be considered as a therapeutic alternative in those patients who are nonadherent, unresponsive or intolerant of oral iron (table 3). Additional indications for parenteral iron preparations, such as functional iron deficiency, require a great deal more study but in theory these agents show great promise. As pediatric trials are lacking in these areas, future studies are badly needed to determine the optimal preparation, dose, infusion strategies, and appropriate patient populations.

References

1 Cogswell ME, Looker AC, Pfeiffer CM, et al: Assessment of iron deficiency in US preschool children and nonpregnant females of childbearing age: National Health and Nutrition Examination Survey 2003–2006. Am J Clin Nutr 2009;89:1334–1342.

2 Ziegler EE: Consumption of cow's milk as a cause of iron deficiency in infants and toddlers. Nutr Rev 2011;69(suppl 1):S37–S42.

3 Goodnough LT, Nemeth E, Ganz T: Detection, evaluation, and management of iron-restricted erythropoiesis. Blood 2010;116:4754–4761.

4 Lozoff B, Georgieff MK: Iron deficiency and brain development. Semin Pediatr Neurol 2006;13:158–165.

5 Lozoff B, Beard J, Connor J, Barbara F, Georgieff M, Schallert T: Long-lasting neural and behavioral effects of iron deficiency in infancy. Nutr Rev 2006; 64:S34–S43; discussion S72–S91.

6 Georgieff MK: Long-term brain and behavioral consequences of early iron deficiency. Nutr Rev 2011; 69(suppl 1):S43–S48.

7 Heeney MM: Anemia. In: Rudolph CD, Rudolph AM, Lister GE, First LR, Gershon AA (eds). Rudolph's Pediatrics, ed 22. New York, McGraw-Hill, 2011, pp 1542–1545.

8 Hallberg L, Ryttinger L, Solvell L: Side-effects of oral iron therapy. A double-blind study of different iron compounds in tablet form. Acta Med Scand Suppl 1966;459:3–10.

9 Chertow GM, Mason PD, Vaage-Nilsen O, Ahlmen J: Update on adverse drug events associated with parenteral iron. Nephrol Dial Transplant 2006;21: 378–382.

10 Chertow GM, Mason PD, Vaage-Nilsen O, Ahlmen J: On the relative safety of parenteral iron formulations. Nephrol Dial Transplant 2004;19: 1571–1575.

11 Pinsk V, Levy J, Moser A, Yerushalmi B, Kapelushnik J: Efficacy and safety of intravenous iron sucrose therapy in a group of children with iron deficiency anemia. Isr Med Assoc J 2008;10:335–338.

12 Crary SE, Hall K, Buchanan GR: Intravenous iron sucrose for children with iron deficiency failing to respond to oral iron therapy. Pediatr Blood Cancer 2011;56:615–619.

13 Auerbach M, Ballard H: Clinical use of intravenous iron: administration, efficacy, and safety. Hematology Am Soc Hematol Educ Program 2010;2010:338–347.

14 Case G: Maintaining iron balance with total-dose infusion of intravenous iron dextran. ANNA J 1998;25: 65–68.

15 Auerbach M, Coyne D, Ballard H: Intravenous iron: from anathema to standard of care. Am J Hematol 2008;83:580–588.

16 Mamula P, Piccoli DA, Peck SN, Markowitz JE, Baldassano RN: Total dose intravenous infusion of iron dextran for iron-deficiency anemia in children with inflammatory bowel disease. J Pediatr Gastroenterol Nutr 2002;34:286–290.

17 Plummer ES, Crary SE, Buchanan GR: Intravenous low molecular weight iron dextran (LMWID) in the treatment of children with iron deficiency anemia (abstract). Pediatr Blood Cancer 2012;521:1026.

18 Auerbach M, Witt D, Toler W, Fierstein M, Lerner RG, Ballard H: Clinical use of the total dose intravenous infusion of iron dextran. J Lab Clin Med 1988; 111:566–570.

19 Auerbach M, Chaudhry M, Goldman H, Ballard H; Value of methylprednisolone in prevention of the arthralgia-myalgia syndrome associated with the total dose infusion of iron dextran: a double blind randomized trial. J Lab Clin Med 1998;131:257–260.

20 Chandler G, Harchowal J, Macdougall IC: Intravenous iron sucrose: establishing a safe dose. Am J Kidney Dis 2001;38:988–991.

21 Fishbane S: Safety issues with iron sucrose. Am J Kidney Dis 2003;41:899; author reply 900.

22 Hassan N, Cahill J, Rajasekaran S, Kovey K: Ferumoxytol infusion in pediatric patients with gastrointestinal disorders: first case series. Ann Pharmacother 2011;45:e63.

23 Rimon E, Kagansky N, Kagansky M, et al: Are we giving too much iron? Low-dose iron therapy is effective in octogenarians. Am J Med 2005;118:1142–1147.
24 Auerbach M: Should intravenous iron be upfront therapy for iron deficiency anemia? Pediatr Blood Cancer 2011;56:511–512.
25 Van Wyck DB, Mangione A, Morrison J, Hadley PE, Jehle JA, Goodnough LT: Large-dose intravenous ferric carboxymaltose injection for iron deficiency anemia in heavy uterine bleeding: a randomized, controlled trial. Transfusion 2009;49:2719–2728.
26 Lee TW, Kolber MR, Fedorak RN, van Zanten SV: Iron replacement therapy in inflammatory bowel disease patients with iron deficiency anemia: a systematic review and meta-analysis. J Crohns Colitis 2012;6:267–275.
27 Cullis JO: Diagnosis and management of anaemia of chronic disease: current status. Br J Haematol 2011; 154:289–300.
28 Steensma DP, Sloan JA, Dakhil SR, et al: Phase III, randomized study of the effects of parenteral iron, oral iron, or no iron supplementation on the erythropoietic response to darbepoetin alfa for patients with chemotherapy-associated anemia. J Clin Oncol 2011;29:97–105.
29 Henry DH: Parenteral iron therapy in cancer-associated anemia. Hematology Am Soc Hematol Educ Program 2010;2010:351–356.
30 Cazzola M, Ponchio L, de Benedetti F, et al: Defective iron supply for erythropoiesis and adequate endogenous erythropoietin production in the anemia associated with systemic-onset juvenile chronic arthritis. Blood 1996;87:4824–4830.

Shelley E. Crary, MD, MSCS
University of Arkansas for Medical Sciences and Arkansas Children's Hospital
1 Children's Way, Slot 512–10
Little Rock, AR 72202 (USA)
E-Mail SECrary@UAMS.edu

Thomas AE, Halsey C (eds): Controversies in Pediatric and Adolescent Hematology.
Pediatr Adolesc Med. Basel, Karger, 2014, vol 17, pp 161–171 (DOI: 10.1159/000350353)

Principles of Transitional Care in Haematology

Paula H.B. Bolton-Maggs[a] · Satarupa Choudhuri[b]

[a]SHOT, Manchester Blood Centre, [b]Manchester Royal Infirmary, Manchester, UK

Abstract

Adolescence (usually defined as aged 10–20 years) is associated with major changes, physical, psychological and social, for the individual and his/her family. Additional difficulties confront the young person with a chronic haematological disease (haemoglobinopathy, bleeding disorder or cancer) who may default from necessary appointments and treatment. This can result in poor outcomes including death. Young people need to transfer to adult services and this is best managed as a supportive process, transition, starting at the age of about 12 years. Transition aims to help the young person become more independent, able to advocate for him/herself and ready for transfer, the time point at which the service provider may change. Young people should be involved in developing their transition plan. Improved education in adolescent issues is required both for paediatricians and adult specialists. There are many models of good practice and there is also evidence that adoption of these results in better outcomes.
Copyright © 2014 S. Karger AG, Basel

Transition refers to the period of time during which a young person moves from dependent childhood to independent adulthood and includes the period of adolescence. In a sense, transition is lifelong but through adolescence in particular, the young person experiences major changes in physical attributes, and in their emotional, social and educational environments as he/she learns to become more independent. This is often a turbulent time both for the individual and his/her family:

> 'I would there were no age between ten and three and twenty, or that youth would sleep out the rest: for there is nothing in the between but getting wenches with child, wronging the ancientry, stealing, fighting' (Shakespeare, from the Winter's Tale as quoted in [1]).

Definitions of adolescence vary but this period usually spans the ages of 10 to about 20 years. Puberty is occurring earlier with many girls now starting menstruation while still in primary school. During adolescence there are changes in brain structure and function which may not be complete in males until their late 20s [2]. Many young person services now recognize this and continue 'transition' beyond the teenage years into the mid-20s or later.

Three sequential stages of normal adolescence are described by Carr-Gregg [3] and captured in three questions facing the young person: 'Who am I?', 'Am I normal?' and 'Where am I going?'. Indeed, the parents and carers may be asking similar questions: 'What's wrong with him?', 'Who does he think he is?' and 'What time will he be home?' [3]. The young person is seeking to discover his/her own identity within the family and the wider social environment including school and society. At the same time as asserting his/her need for greater independence, however, the young person is still more fragile and vulnerable than he/she may appear.

These changes impact on medical care. In the same way that the young person may challenge his/her family values and structure and indulge in exploratory and risk-taking behaviour, so he/she may challenge the medical authority figures as he/she seeks independence. The young person may become less compliant with both clinic attendance and with necessary therapy, and the nature of the relationship between the medical staff and the young person will change. This needs to be recognized and sympathetically managed. In general, the management of medical conditions in childhood is determined by the parents with the medical staff, but in adults, directly with the individual who usually attends on his/her own. Those with chronic or lifelong conditions such as haemoglobin disorders or haemophilia will need to make the transition, which will frequently mean not only a change in medical personnel whom they have known perhaps since early childhood, but also to a different clinical environment or a different hospital. It is notable that today's young people increasingly communicate electronically, searching the internet for information rather than asking an adult for it, and using social media in ways that many adults do not. This should be kept in mind when we attempt to provide information for them.

How can we optimize transition?

Recognition of the Risks

The number of young people aged 10–19 in the UK has increased over the past two decades to more than 7.5 million. Although youth is usually perceived as healthy, emergency admissions in the 16- to 19-year age group have increased significantly [4]. With improvements in medical care, an increasing number of young people with chronic conditions are surviving into adult life, for example 85% of children now treated with surgery for congenital heart disease will reach adulthood, and there are increasing numbers of adult survivors of cystic fibrosis, diabetes and chronic kidney diseases. While this is good news, the bad news is that there is evidence that a failure of joined up care results in poor outcomes [5]. A UK study of transition for renal transplant recipients reported that at 36 months after transfer to adult care, more than a third of young people had lost their transplants. However, this can be significantly improved by introduction of an integrated transition service [6]. Failure to follow up congenital heart disease patients was associated with an increased risk of adverse outcomes (the development of additional cardiac abnormalities requiring urgent intervention) [7]. With respect to haematological disorders, the life expectancy for haemophilia in developed countries now approaches that of the normal population; children with haemoglobin disorders often survive into adulthood, and there are many more survivors than in the past from paediatric cancers. Not only may there not be adult physicians with experience to manage these young adults (e.g. grown-up patients with congenital heart disease or biochemical disorders) but also society contains an increasing number of young people requiring medical care for actual or potential disabilities which in turn affect their educational and social needs. In addition to those children with ongoing chronic illness, children who have survived cancer and who are in long-term remission or cured also have particular needs. There may be other long-term health problems related to late side effects of treatment, including fertility issues [8] which need to be addressed. These issues have been explored by Nathan et al. [9] noting that 'for those fortunate patients who survive their cancer, the period of survivorship will comprise the longest portion of their cancer journey'. In addition to the physical and emotional changes of adolescence, this is a time when young people are making important decisions about careers, when they need good support from both family and in the health-care setting. In a recent consultation on youth in the UK [10], a discussion paper on 'adolescent brain development' was found to be very useful in helping parents, educationalists and potentially health care personnel to be more aware and understanding of the major changes in neuronal connections taking place which may not be complete until well into the third decade. The subsequent UK initiative, the 'Children and Young People's Health Outcomes Forum' published its report in 2012 [11] with issues identified by the young people ('no decision about me without me') at the centre. The authors noted that 'too many health outcomes for children and young people are poor, and for many this is involved with failures in care'. The report noted that many clinical staff have inadequate training in paediatrics and child health. That adult physicians and paediatricians have little or no training in adolescent medicine has been noted before [12]. The forum recommends some new indicators for inclusion within the NHS outcomes framework including 'effective transition from children's to adult services' and 'age-appropriate services with particular reference to teenagers'. It is important to involve young people in decisions about transition services. Despite recent emphasis on involvement of young people in their own health care, a review [13] of 38 surveys performed by the UK National Health Service found that patients under 16 years of age were very rarely included (<0.6% of over 10 million respondents) and young adults aged 16–24 years reported a lower level of satisfaction than older adults. Much of this is not new, but it has proved difficult to put into practice. Improving training in adolescent issues has begun to be addressed in at least two ways in the UK. Firstly, the

Royal College of Paediatrics and Child Health in association with the Royal College of General Practitioners has developed an e-learning package on adolescent health with 70 interactive sessions covering 30 topics including training on disability and transition (funded by the Department of Health and available at http://www.e-lfh.org.uk/projects/ah/index.html). This is free for all healthcare professionals within the National Health Service. Secondly, a multidisciplinary group of interested specialists is working within the Royal College of Physicians (London) to consider what can be done to improve care for young adults. One fruit from this has been the inclusion of core topics concerning adolescent health into curricula for physician training [4].

Particular Issues for Adolescents

In the paediatric setting, the young person is on firm ground receiving coordinated care across different medical specialties from a multidisciplinary team that knows the patient well. The transfer to the adult sector is often into the unknown, where there may be limited expertise in the adult service either because the care is not focused on the needs of young people or the condition is so rare. Transition can be defined as the 'purposeful, planned movement of adolescents and young adults with chronic physical and medical conditions from child-centered to adult-orientated health care systems' [14] and ensures that their care will remain both medically and developmentally appropriate. Transition is a process, transfer is an event. A number of steps are now recommended to ensure that 'transition' is a process of adaptation, while 'transfer' is the date when the young person moves from one healthcare environment to the other. The timing of transfer may be related to rules or laws, such as the age limit for admission to a paediatric unit, which will vary with unit but generally be 18 years, or another convenient event such as entering tertiary education. Transfer can be preceded by informal meetings to introduce the young person and his/her parents to the adult staff and setting. This is very helpful. Transition may be more difficult for the parents than for the adolescent, and parents often need help to 'let go'. They also need to feel confident with the new arrangements. While children's care usually or often involves their family, including parents and sometimes siblings, adult care does not. Adults usually attend on their own and may feel inhibited from bringing a supporter into the consultation with them which is unfortunate. This is reflected in a survey of transition literature [15] where the authors noted one study [16] where 70% of providers serving children and adolescents expected the young person to be seen with the parent or guardian but 67% adult providers expected the patient to be seen on his/her own. This is a culture in adult medicine which needs changing. The manner in which this supportive care is transferred to the adult healthcare system is crucial to the continuing wellbeing of the young person and their willingness to continue and comply with health support and treatment. Thus, the goal of transition for young adults with special health care needs is to maximize lifelong functioning and potential through the provision of high-quality, developmentally appropriate health care services that continue uninterrupted as the individual moves from adolescence to adulthood.

Good practice starts with early discussion of the fact of transition and possible transfer, and includes preparation of a written transition plan, with goals to be achieved by specific dates. In the past, transfer has occurred without adequate transition, with very little information handover between medical staff other than the bare medical facts. The new team needs more than this including information about the psychological and social needs of the young person, and information about their educational and vocational aspirations, in other words an appreciation of the whole person. Preparation can begin at about 12 years of age and continue throughout the next years. This is a good time to offer the young person the opportunity to be seen on his/her own for at least part of any consultation, to discuss his/her own contribution to managing his/her chronic disease. For example, in haemophilia, a boy can learn to administer his own factor replacement before the age of 10 years, and should be encouraged to take responsibility for this, including knowing when it is required and completing his treatment records. Discussion can take place about who accompanies the young person at the new consultations (if anyone). After transfer, as far as possible young people should have continuity of care, seeing the same doctor, with a restricted number of people at the consultation for instance not be seen by a different junior doctor at each visit in the adult sector, or to be faced with a room full of medical students.

Models of Transition

There is no single 'right answer' to effective transition. While the key principles are established, different hospitals can achieve these in different ways.

Key principles are:

(a) Recognition that this is a process not an event.

(b) Start discussion with the young person early, by age 12, and note that the program needs to be individualized.

(c) Map out specific goals in the different areas of the young person's life.

(d) The transition program should be established by the paediatric and adult teams working together with a written shared policy.

(e) Both teams should seek input or training in adolescent issues.

(f) The transition plan must also address the needs of the parents/guardians who may find it hard to let go.

(g) The young person should collaborate in the process and thus enhance his/her sense of control and independence. This is likely to require a trusted key adult as an advocate, who will be particularly helpful for the first few appointments in the adult sector. Adult physicians will underestimate the extent to which adolescents are not yet able to advocate for themselves, usually having had no training and no experience in the use of the adult health systems.

Where care of a chronic condition continues in the same hospital throughout life, the team members need to ensure that the young person is encouraged to be seen on his/her own, to learn to make his/her own decisions and to establish different types of relationships. The young man may not feel able to talk about his sexuality to a nurse who has known him since infancy. It may be difficult then to have the freedom to discuss sexuality, drugs or other adolescent issues. These may be uncomfortable for discussion with both paediatric and adult staff whose focus is the medical specialty; in this case the young person will benefit from access to appropriate staff. Goldenring [17] has noted that 'for teenagers, a psychosocial review is at least as important as the physical exam'. A systematic method for interviewing in this way includes HEEADSSS, i.e. Home environment, Education and employment, Eating, peer-related Activities, Drugs, Sexuality, Suicide/depression and Safety from injury and violence [17].

Different models are possible. Where the young person will continue to be seen in the same hospital, transition may appear to be easier since the staff caring for him/her may not change; where adult physicians are introduced it is easier to do this in a staged manner. However, transition is necessary for the staff as well as the young person, and the need to introduce other members of staff must be recognized. It is not always healthy for a whole family (for example with a bleeding disorder) to be seen together. While this may seem a good arrangement, each individual will have needs and issues which require privacy with assurance that confidentiality will be maintained. In adult practice this tends to be assumed by doctor and patient, but it is particularly important for adolescents to be reassured of this, since their experience is that the parents are told everything (sometimes over their heads!). This is also an opportunity for the young person to develop his/her own advocacy skills and learn to be seen alone. A continual challenge faced by the health care provider during adolescence is of negotiating the balance between advocating for the young person and remaining inclusive of parents.

Some hospitals have specific arrangements for adolescent clinics and physicians with training, but this tends to be the minority. A period of joint clinics with both adult and paediatric specialists together with specialist nurses enables the young person and his family to establish the new relationships. In addition, it is good for the patient and his/her family to make an informal visit to the new centre, to learn about how it works and what the contact mechanisms are in advance of the transfer event.

Transition: Experience in Haematological Disorders

Transition is an essential part of growing up for all children with genetic haematological disorders (haemoglobinopathies, bleeding disorders, constitutional bone marrow failure, congenital haemolysis) and particularly for children who survive cancer, and those who are diagnosed and are undergoing treatment (including those with uncertain outlook) through their adolescent years.

Survival into adult life has been the norm in haemophilia for several decades in developed countries where replacement therapy has been readily available since the 1970s and prophylaxis has become more commonplace in the last two decades. As a result, many boys with haemophilia have normal or near normal joints, have no disability and appear very little different from their peers, to the extent that they also may feel 'invincible'. Haemophilia care has devolved to specialist centres. While some boys with severe haemophilia learn increasing independence from below 10 years of age, when they learn to self-infuse, they have the same needs as other adolescents in transition. Moreover the degree of independence is extremely variable with some young adults in their late teens still dependent on a parent for infusion. A good comprehensive transition program has been developed by the National Hemophilia Foundation in the USA which can be adapted for use elsewhere. The principles can also be adapted for other disorders. This recognizes that transition starts early (at diagnosis) and continues into adult life [18]. The guidelines identify five different age groups, birth to 4 years, 5–8 years, 9–12 years, 13–15 years and 16–18 years. Goals and objectives, and strategies to meet them, are discussed under different headings including social support, health and lifestyles, educational/vocational/financial planning, self-advocacy and self-esteem, independent health care behaviours and sexual health. This comprehensive program may be locally adapted. In recent years there has been increasing recognition of the importance of managing adolescence with the publication from the Department of Health (DH) of national transition guidelines in the UK [19] followed by 'welcome' criteria that hospitals should adopt in order to become more young person-friendly [20]. However, the lack of knowledge about these guidelines among professionals who manage young adults is disappointing. In a UK survey (2010) of haemophilia centre directors, fewer than half knew of these documents (only 9/28 (32%) centre directors were aware of the DH national guidelines, and only 12/28 (43%) were aware of the 'you're welcome' quality criteria).

Surveys of treatment adherence in haemophilia demonstrate a fall-off in adolescence [21] when young people want to be like their peers and not bothered with the inconvenience of regular prophylaxis, for example. An additional worry now that prophylaxis is so effective in preventing joint bleeds and disability is that young men underestimate the significance of their bleeding disorder and the danger posed by injuries, particularly since many will never have experienced a significant bleed. A recent study consulted 30 boys (15 aged 10–16 years) from a single paediatric centre where prophylaxis starts early and is tailored to the individual so that daily dosing may be appropriate, particularly for those participating in sports. Regular daily dosing, or regimes designed in close consultation with the boy rather than imposed by health care professionals, was associated with better self-management and positive attitudes towards their disorder [22]. This is an instructive lesson in the importance of involving young people in their treatment decisions.

Similar adherence issues exist for young people on parenteral chelation therapy for thalassaemia major [23] where iron overload continues to be a significant cause of morbidity and death [24, 25]. UK guidelines on the management of thalassaemia detail the standards for transition including the general principles described above, and suggest that a transition plan is started by the age of 13 years, also noting that the time of transfer should be flexible [26].

The literature on transition in haemoglobin disorders has been reviewed [15] however only five of the 17 studies considered related to haemoglobinopathies. The three main obstacles to transition that emerged were firstly a lack of transitional support i.e. no resources, no time and no personnel and difficulty finding a suitable adult provider, secondly limited transition programs and thirdly resistance to transition toward adult health care. Resistance to transition by young people and their carers can be substantially reduced by a good transition program. The young person wants to remain in the familiar environment, particularly when unwell, and this can result in these 'adults' being admitted to the paediatric centres despite 'transfer'. An Australian study reported that 47% of adults admitted to the paediatric hospital with severe complications of their chronic disorders (endocrine, neurological or oncological) over a 10-year period were those who had been transferred to adult care [27]. If transition is not satisfactory the patient is likely to return the paediatric provider or paediatric emergency department. A survey of 14 adolescents with sickle cell disease from a single centre [28] identified a number of common themes for the patients: firstly 'I don't want to go' – associated with sadness, apprehension, fear of the unknown, a sense of being abandoned by their paediatric team. The second theme was 'What's going to happen to me?' – several participants had received notification of transfer at inappropriate times such as at a visit to the emergency department near their 18th birthday. They were given a list of adult providers and told to make an appointment. The third theme was the sense of being pushed into adult care without adequate preparations and finally 'accepting that I had to leave'. Another study assessed 70 patients with sickle cell disease at a single centre and demonstrated poor readiness for transition although recognizing its inevitability [29].

Young people with cancer and cancer survivors face additional issues. Young cancer survivors may have little knowledge of their original diagnosis and treatment; late effects from therapy may be unexpected. Transition for these young people will therefore include patient education and other steps outlined in figure 1 [9]. The issues facing these young people, and models for their care, are discussed in a useful review from Canada [9]. Teenagers with cancer may be more fortunate than other young people with chronic disease as there has been recognition of their need for dedicated inpatient facilities, a place of their own in hospital. The Teenage Cancer Trust in the UK is a charity devoted to improving the lives of teenagers and young adults with cancer and lists 20 hospitals in the UK with dedicated inpatient facilities for teenagers – the aim is to keep life as normal as possible, and 'the young person first, cancer patient second' (see www.cancerteenagetrust.org). Many general hospitals would benefit from facilities dedicated to young people in this way, and the number of young people using emergency facilities and requiring inpatient admission would justify this in many large centres, but to date this has not been part of hospital development apart from cancer management. The development of long-term follow-up of paediatric cancer survivors

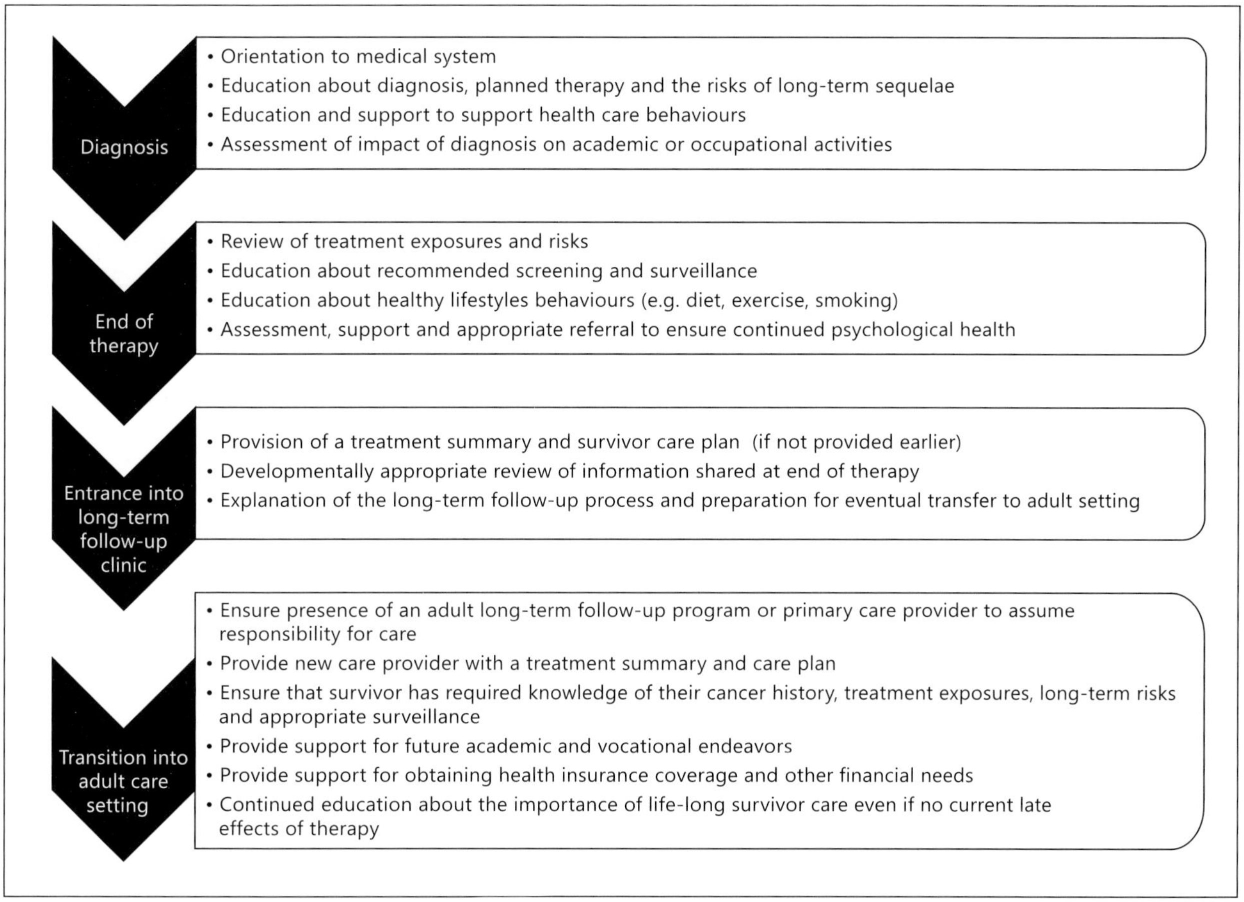
Diagnosis
• Orientation to medical system
• Education about diagnosis, planned therapy and the risks of long-term sequelae
• Education and support to support health care behaviours
• Assessment of impact of diagnosis on academic or occupational activities
End of therapy
• Review of treatment exposures and risks
• Education about recommended screening and surveillance
• Education about healthy lifestyles behaviours (e.g. diet, exercise, smoking)
• Assessment, support and appropriate referral to ensure continued psychological health
Entrance into long-term follow-up clinic
• Provision of a treatment summary and survivor care plan (if not provided earlier)
• Developmentally appropriate review of information shared at end of therapy
• Explanation of the long-term follow-up process and preparation for eventual transfer to adult setting
Transition into adult care setting
• Ensure presence of an adult long-term follow-up program or primary care provider to assume responsibility for care
• Provide new care provider with a treatment summary and care plan
• Ensure that survivor has required knowledge of their cancer history, treatment exposures, long-term risks and appropriate surveillance
• Provide support for future academic and vocational endeavors
• Provide support for obtaining health insurance coverage and other financial needs
• Continued education about the importance of life-long survivor care even if no current late effects of therapy

Fig. 1. Key steps in the multiple transitions from cancer diagnosis to long-term follow-up in an adult care setting [9].

has been reviewed [30] noting that there is an increasing number, estimated at 1 in 570 persons aged 20–40 years. These individuals are at risk of long-term complications from their treatment, perhaps 25–40%, and require appropriate long-term follow-up. Some paediatric cancers are unknown in adults meaning that adult physicians may not be adequately equipped to monitor the late effects. In some centres this has been overcome by the paediatric oncologist attending a transition or young adult clinic in the adult centre to facilitate knowledge as well as providing overlap and continuity of care. These young survivors may well require detailed information about their disease and its treatment, which may have taken place at an early age when the child was not able to understand and retain information that will be required later in life.

A general review of the literature on adherence after transition including 12 papers, none haematological (6 in diabetes, 4 solid organ transplants and 2 respiratory diseases) [31], confirmed poor adherence to medical appointments and oral medications which translated into adverse outcomes (including death). The introduction of a 'transition coordinator' to remind patients of their appointments and to conduct guidance discussions in two studies led to improved outcomes.

These findings reinforce the need to develop proper transition programs so the young person is prepared to move on, has confidence in the new staff who he/she has had a chance to get to know, and that this process has involved helping the parents/carers to accept the change.

It is important to consider whether transition programs are effective. A systematic literature review in 2010 examined studies which evaluated health outcomes. Of 10 studies meeting the inclusion criteria, 6 (all in diabetes) demonstrated statistically significant improvements in outcomes [5]. These studies were heterogeneous, but common themes were patient education, transition coordinators and specific transition clinics.

Conclusion

It is clear that insufficient attention has been given to the major issues confronting young people with chronic disorders as they move through adolescence. Paediatricians and adult specialists need to work more closely together to make the journey easier for both the patients and their parents. Useful models are now available, and there is evidence that good shared care with better handover is associated with better and safer outcomes.

References

1 RCPCH: Bridging the Gaps. Health care for adolescents. http://www.rcpch.ac.uk/system/files/protected/page/bridging_the_gaps.pdf 2003.
2 Steinberg L: A behavioral scientist looks at the science of adolescent brain development. Brain Cogn 2010;72:160–164.
3 Carr-Gregg M: Surviving Adolescents. London, Penguin, 2005.
4 McDonagh JE, Robinson AJ: Growing up: the role of the Royal College of Physicians. Clin Med 2012;12:197–199.
5 Crowley R, Wolfe I, Lock K, McKee M: Improving the transition between paediatric and adult healthcare: a systematic review. Arch Dis Child 2011;96:548–553.
6 Harden PN, Walsh G, Bandler N, Bradley S, Lonsdale D, Taylor J, Marks SD: Bridging the gap: an integrated paediatric to adult clinical service for young adults with kidney failure. BMJ 2012;344:e3718.
7 Yeung E, Kay J, Roosevelt GE, Brandon M, Yetman AT: Lapse of care as a predictor for morbidity in adults with congenital heart disease. Int J Cardiol 2008;125:62–65.
8 Henderson TO, Friedman DL, Meadows AT: Childhood cancer survivors: transition to adult-focused risk-based care. Pediatr 2010;126:129–136.
9 Nathan PC, Hayes-Lattin B, Sisler JJ, Hudson MM: Critical issues in transition and survivorship for adolescents and young adults with cancers. Cancer 2011;117(10 suppl):2335–2341.
10 Her Majesty's Government: Positive for Youth. Department of Education. http://media.education.gov.uk/assets/files/positive%20for%20youth.pdf 2011.
11 Lewis E, Lenehan C: Report of the Children and Young People's Health Outcomes Forum. http://dh.gov.uk/health/files/2012/07/cyp.report.pdf 2012.
12 McDonagh JE, Minnaar G, Kelly K, O'Connor D, Shaw KL: Unmet education and training needs in adolescent health of health professionals in a UK children's hospital. Acta Paediatr 2006;95:715–719.
13 Hargreaves DS, Viner RM: Children's and young people's experience of the National Health Service in England: a review of national surveys 2001–2011. Arch Dis Child 2012;97:661–666.

14 Blum RW, Garell D, Hodgman CH, Jorissen TW, Okinow NA, Orr DP, Slap GB: Transition from child-centered to adult health-care systems for adolescents with chronic conditions. A position paper of the Society for Adolescent Medicine. J Adolesc Health 1993;14:570–576.
15 Bryant R, Walsh T: Transition of the chronically ill youth with hemoglobinopathy to adult health care: an integrative review of the literature. J Pediatr Health 2009;23:37–48.
16 Telfair J, Alexander LR, Loosier PS, Alleman-Velez PL, Simmons J: Providers' perspectives and beliefs regarding transition to adult care for adolescents with sickle cell disease. J Health Care Poor Underserved 2004;15:443–461.
17 Goldenring J: Getting into adolescent heads: an essential update. Contemp Pediatr 2004;21:64.
18 MASAC: Transition Guidelines for People with Bleeding Disorders (MASAC Document #147). http://hemophilia.org/NHFWeb/MainPgs/MainNHF.aspx?menuid=contentid=2072003.
19 UK Department of Health: Transition – Getting it Right for Young People. http://www.dh.gov.uk/prod_consum_dh/groups/dh_digitalassets/@dh/@en/documents/digitalasset/dh_4132149.pdf 2006.
20 UK Department of Health: You're Welcome Quality criteria for young people friendly health services. http://www.dh.gov.uk/prod_consum_dh/groups/dh_digitalassets/documents/digitalasset/dh_127632.pdf 2011.
21 Breakey VR, Blanchette VS, Bolton-Maggs PH: Towards comprehensive care in transition for young people with haemophilia. Haemophilia 2010;16:848–857.
22 Khair K, Gibson F, Meerabeau L: The benefits of prophylaxis: views of adolescents with severe haemophilia. Haemophilia 2012;18:e286–e289.
23 Porter JB, Evangeli M, El-Beshlawy A: Challenges of adherence and persistence with iron chelation therapy. Int J Hematol 2011;94:453–460.
24 Rashid M, Karimi M: Compliance of deferoxamine injection in beta-thalassaemia major patients in Iran. Transfus Med 2012;22:104–107.
25 Modell B, Khan M, Darlison M: Survival in beta-thalassaemia major in the UK: data from the UK Thalassaemia Register. Lancet 2000;355:2051–2052.
26 UK-Thalassaemia-Society: Standards for the clinical care of children and adults with thalassaemia in the UK. http://www.ukts.org/pdfs/awareness/standards2008.pdf pp 47–48.
27 Lam PY, Fitzgerald BB, Sawyer SM: Young adults in children's hospitals: why are they there? Med J Aus 2005;182:381–384.
28 Bryant R, Young A, Cesario S, Binder B: Transition of chronically ill youth to adult health care: experience of youth with hemoglobinopathy. J Pediatr Health Care 2011;25:275–283.
29 McPherson M, Thaniel L, Minniti CP: Transition of patients with sickle cell disease from pediatric to adult care: assessing patient readiness. Pediatr Blood Cancer 2009;52:838–841.
30 Ginsberg JP, Hobbie WL, Carlson CA, Meadows AT: Delivering long-term follow-up care to pediatric cancer survivors: transitional care issues. Pediatr Blood Cancer 2006;46:169–173.
31 Pai A, Ostendorf HM: Treatment adherence in adolescents and young adults affected by chronic illness during the health care transition from pediatric to adult health care: a literature review. Children's Health Care 2011;40:16–33.

Dr. Paula Bolton-Maggs
SHOT
Manchester Blood Centre, Plymouth Grove
Manchester M13 9LL (UK)
E-Mail paula.bolton-maggs@manchester.ac.uk

Author Index

Subject Index